PHENOMENOLOGY AND TREATMENT OF
PSYCHOSEXUAL DISORDERS

PHENOMENOLOGY AND TREATMENT OF PSYCHOSEXUAL DISORDERS

edited by

William E. Fann, M.D.
Ismet Karacan, M.D. (Med) D. Sci.
Alex D. Pokorny, M.D.
Robert L. Williams, M.D.

all of the

Department of Psychiatry
Baylor College of Medicine
Houston, Texas

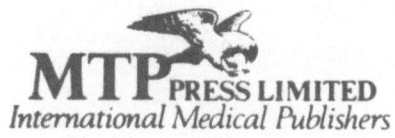
MTP PRESS LIMITED
International Medical Publishers

Published in the UK and Europe by
MTP Press Limited
Falcon House
Lancaster, England

Published in the US by
SPECTRUM PUBLICATIONS, INC.
175-20 Wexford Terrace
Jamaica, NY 11432

ISBN-13: 978-94-011-6328-6   e-ISBN-13: 978-94-011-6326-2
DOI: 10.1007/978-94-011-6326-2

Foreword

This is the sixth in a series of volumes sponsored by the Department of Psychiatry of Baylor College of Medicine, each reviewing one broad category of psychiatric disorders. Earlier conferences have focused on well-established psychiatric categories such as depression, schizophrenia, and alcoholism. Psychosexual disorders are usually considered as a subgroup of psychiatric disorders, and form one of the major categories of the DSM-III Classification of Mental Disorders. However, psychosexual disorders are also of concern to all physicians and clinicians, working in virtually every field of medicine.

The whole area of human sexuality has been characterized by rapid advances during the last few decades. Notable contributions have been from psychoanalysis, from the work of Kinsey and associates, and particularly from the work of Masters and Johnson, which has led to new stress on psychosexual *dysfunctions,* in addition to the earlier interest in paraphilias, gender identity disorders, etc. Still later there has been increasing emphasis on disorders of sexual desire.

A further step in this trend to more effective treatment based on more valid knowledge is the work presented in the chapter by Karacan, Aslan, and Williams. They stress, in their discussion of the differential diagnosis of impotence, the weakness of an exclusive dependence on patients' reports. They propose that diagnostic evaluation in this area must include specialized physical and physiological examinations so that the patient's problem of inadequate erection is established by direct examination. They recommend comparable direct evaluations of other psychosexual disorders, and caution that without such data evaluations of treatment must remain somewhat speculative.

This volume presents discussions of current knowledge and opinion in a broad array of topics related to psychosexual disorders. Several chapters deal with the etiology and development of psychosexual disorders. Schweitzer and Brown review the role of long-continued use of alcohol in development of sexual dysfunction, as well as the role of acute intoxication in sex and violence, as in rape. Dr. Socarides presents a detailed historical review of psychoanalytic views regarding the etiology and development of homosexuality. Dr. Krueger presents a lucid exposition of gender dysphoria, including very clear definitions and delimitations. Meyer and Dupkin present a detailed interpretation of the development and dynamics of sado-masochism.

Community and social aspects of psychosexual disorders are reviewed, including a thoughtful and philosophical review of pornography by Morris Lipton, based in part on his experience on the President's Commission on Pornography. This includes an interesting review of the legal status and the role of public attitudes in this area. Betsy Comstock reviews the topic of abortion, including psychodynamic aspects and implications. Domeena Renshaw provides a wide-ranging review of the topic of incest in which she points out that this behavior is much more common than usually assumed. She also provides many practical suggestions on clinical management, family dynamics, and legal issues. Dr. Richard Rada presents a comprehensive discussion of rape, stressing that the crime is based in psychological experiences of power and control. Dr. Cantrell has written a scholarly review of the place of sexual education in the training of physicians and presents results of a study of medical students' knowledge of sex and sexuality, with some surprising findings. Dr. James Lomax considers the importance of this training in psychiatric residency programs and suggests a model for a goal-oriented approach to the education of new psychiatrists in diagnosing and treating psychosexual disorders.

The volume also includes helpful chapters on clinical procedures, with Dr. Lauro Halstead's sensitive and perceptive chapter on sexual adjustment of the handicapped, with specific suggestions for any physician treating patients with severe physical limitations, noting in particular the therapeutic alliance with affectionate and adaptable partners of afflicted patients.

Together these chapters constitute an updating of a great many aspects of psychosexual disorders, including clarification of when and where they exist, how and when they may be treated, and how the physician may be prepared for his or her role in this arena. The material here supplements the widely published descriptive and therapeutic work of such major contributors to the field as Masters and Johnson, Helen Singer Kaplan, and Robert Stoller, and, in an area of medical concern as much affected by changing cultural climates as by emerging scientific information, is intended to suggest the state of the art at the beginning of the 1980s.

William E. Fann, M.D.
Ismet Karacan, M.D., D Sc. (Med.)
Alex D. Pokorny, M.D.
Robert L. Williams, M.D.

Contributors

Cenzig Aslan, M.D. • Post-Doctoral Fellow, Department of Psychiatry, Baylor College of Medicine, Houston, Texas

Eleanor Brown, B.A. • Inpatient Director, Alcoholism Treatment Unit, The Methodist Hospital, Houston, Texas

William A. Cantrell, M.D. • Professor of Psychiatry, Baylor College of Medicine, Houston, Texas

Betsy S. Comstock, M.D. • Associate Professor of Psychiatry, Baylor College of Medicine, *and* Director, Day Hospital, Veterans Administration Medical Center, Houston, Texas

Carol Dupkin, B.A. • Assistant in Psychiatry, Johns Hopkins University School of Medicine, *and* Research Coordinator, Consultation Unit, The Johns Hopkins Medical Institutions, Baltimore, Maryland

William E. Fann, M.D. • Professor of Psychiatry, Associate Professor of Pharmacology, Baylor College of Medicine, *and* Chief, Psychiatry Service, Veterans Administration Medical Center, Houston, Texas

Lauro S. Halstead, M.D. • Associate Professor, Departments of Rehabilitation, Physical Medicine, and Community Medicine, Baylor College of Medicine, *and* Attending Physician, The Institute for Rehabilitation and Research, Houston, Texas

Ismet Karacan, M.D., DSc. (Med) • Professor of Psychiatry, Baylor College of Medicine, *and* Associate Chief of Staff for Research, Veterans Administration Medical Center, Houston, Texas

David W. Krueger, M.D. • Associate Professor of Psychiatry, Baylor College of Medicine, *and* Director, Baylor Adult Outpatient Psychiatric Clinic, Houston, Texas

Morris A. Lipton, M.D., Ph.D. • Kenan Professor of Psychiatry, University of North Carolina School of Medicine, Chapel Hill, North Carolina

James W. Lomax, M.D. • Assistant Professor of Psychiatry, *and* Director of Psychiatric Residency Training, Baylor College of Medicine, Houston, Texas

Jon K. Meyer, M.D. • Associate Professor of Psychiatry, The Johns Hopkins School of Medicine, *and* Director, Consultation Unit, The Johns Hopkins Medical Institutions, Baltimore, Maryland

Alex D. Pokorny, M.D. • Professor and Vice Chairman, Department of Psychiatry, Baylor College of Medicine, Houston, Texas

Richard T. Rada, M.D. • Professor and Vice Chairman, Department of Psychiatry, University of New Mexico School of Medicine, Albuquerque, New Mexico

Domeena C. Renshaw, M.B., Ch.B. (UCT), M.D. • Professor of Psychiatry, Loyola University of Chicago, Maywood, Illinois

Laurence R. Schweitzer, M.D. • Associate Professor of Psychiatry, Baylor College of Medicine, *and* Deputy Chief of Psychiatry, The Methodist Hospital, Houston, Texas

Charles W. Socarides, M.D. • Professor of Psychiatry, Downstate Medical Center, New York, New York

Charles Tirrell, M.S. • Director, Outpatient Alcoholism Services, The Methodist Hospital, Houston, Texas

Robert L. Williams, M.D. • D.C. and Irene Ellwood Professor and Chairman, Department of Psychiatry, Baylor College of Medicine, Houston, Texas

Table of Contents

PHENOMENOLOGY AND TREATMENT OF PSYCHOSEXUAL DISORDERS

Understanding and Treating Incest

Domeena C. Renshaw

INTRODUCTION

What specific acts constitute incest? Who commits incest? How can the psychiatric literature help us to understand and treat patients who present with questions and problems concerning sexualized affection in the family?

The first surprise is that Diagnostic and Statistical Manual of Mental Disorders I, II, and III do not mention the word incest at all. Secondly, there is the professional realization that the way incest presents to a psychiatrist, quite often incidentally in history-taking, is usually different from the way the family physician may be confronted, which is mostly in crises of pregnancy or incestuous rape. Third, the definition of incest is incomplete, resulting in academic and clinical confusion, which of course raises doubts about the usefulness and accuracy of conclusions drawn from researchers who make a special search for incest participants.

Incest may or may not involve a child; it may or may not be coercive or abusive; it may or may not be coital.

The proper place to begin, therefore, is with a definition of terms. The meaning of incest is determined by the frame of reference in which the term is applied; it is appropriate to define the term in accordance with the purposes to which it is to be put. Specific frames of reference are: legal, moral-religious, sociological, anthropological, biological-genetic, and psychological. Incest may mean something different *between* contexts as well as having a variety of meanings *within* each particular context.

1

An unconsummated desire to have sexual relations with a close blood relative may have moral-religious and psychological implications and be considered incestuous, though from a legal or biological-genetic standpoint it would not be so judged. Or a sociologist studying Israeli kibbutzim may note the rarity of intermarriage among young people in the same kibbutz and inaccurately deduce that this proves the existence of an "incest taboo," though in principle such marriages are not thought of as incestuous in any other than a psychological frame of reference.

In a psychological frame of reference, incest is identified as a problem by the affected individual. In the other frames of reference mentioned (legal, moral, biological, sociological), incest is specified as a problem by nonpersonally affected legislators, clergy, teachers, or counselors. Thus, it is possible that "incest" can be a problem for the individual and not for society; it may be a problem for society but not for the individual; or it may be a problem for both the individual and society.

Further, a problem might develop for an isolated incest-accepting family from the hills of Puerto Rico, Mexico, or the Appalachians when incest is discovered and made known to the larger culture. Or, for the involved individual, problems may arise from discovery, rejection, and stigmatization rather than from the sexual contact itself. Clear formulation and definition of terms are therefore essential to understand and deal adequately with the question of incest, either clinically or academically.

PRESENT KNOWLEDGE

Incest may present in three ways: (1) as a crisis (often child-adult), (2) incidentally (as when an adult or teen reports past personal history), (3) by special search, as in a study of incest participants.

Incest evokes strong emotions which may be categorized as: (1) avoidance—recoil, withdrawal, silence, fear, anxiety; (2) attack—moral outrage, "taboo," violence, death sentence; (3) attraction—arousal, interest.

THE PROBLEM OF DEFINITION

Essential perspectives from which to discuss incest are: (1) biological-genetic, (2) sociological-anthropological, (3) moral-religious, (4) legal, and (5) psychosocial (Renshaw and Renshaw, 1977).

Biological-Genetic

The biological-genetic approach does not deal with the morality or legality of incest; it objectively considers the results of inbreeding. Negative results have been somewhat exaggerated. The quality of the initial gene pool is as important as the closeness of kinship. Agricultural pedigree inbreeding deliberately concentrates positive characteristics, with the usual results being some superior, a few inferior, and most (80 percent) average. Deleterious consequences may occur for the affected 10 percent or less. However, some of these do not survive, and the larger population is thus "cleansed" of undesirable genes. A few available reports of incestuous offspring in the medical literature (healthy children are not reported on) have not emphasized non-incest-related risk factors such as poor antenatal care, attempted abortion, mental retardation of incest partners (initial gene pool), and the very young age of the mothers.

Existence of an "inborn" (biological) anti-incest instinct has been postulated but has not withstood scientific scrutiny or anthropological data.

Sociological-Anthropological

Sociological-anthropological studies reveal that attitudes toward and practice of incest vary widely cross-culturally (Ford and Beach, 1970). Ancient Egyptian, Roman, and Polynesian brother-sister, even mother-son, marriages were accepted for the aristocracy. Some contemporary primitive and literate groups mandate first cousin marriages while others forbid unions not only within consanguineous family but also within "classificatory" kinships, so that sometimes an entire village may be considered sexually and maritally out-of-bounds, with violations judged incestuous. Bondings for consolidation of property and for survival have been theorized to explain why incest was condoned, but also why it was prohibited. As mentioned, some social anthropologists have cited the Israeli kibbutz as a model of closed group behavior that simulates a family: they claim the close childhood rearing fosters a "natural (romantic) aversion," mandating that kibbutz peers do not mate. This claim is exaggerated; such marriages do occur (Cohen, 1978).

Penalties for incest vary cross-culturally and range from the death sentence to expiatory offerings, fines, imprisonment, or social ostracism without other criminal punishment.

What does become clear from a study of groups of people in the past and present is that incest never was and still is not an absolute or universal taboo, as has been incorrectly stated and too often repeated in academic literature.

Moral-Religious

Religion evaluates incest in moral-ethical terms. According to the Judeo-Christian tradition, incest is a sinful contravention of God's law. However, the religious definition of incest has changed over time. For instance, the Roman Catholic Church once classified sexual relations between two persons of the seventh degree of kinship and between two witnesses of the baptism of a child (spiritual relatives) as forbidden, sinful, and incestuous. Currently, marriage between first cousins requires a relatively easily-obtained dispensation from a Chancery Office.

Legal

Legally, incest is stipulated by statute as a criminal act, though the definition varies with the jurisdiction. In most of the United States, sexual intercourse or marriage between blood (consanguineous) relatives of first cousin kinship or closer is defined as incest and considered a felony. An Illinois priest (or other marriage officer) may not by law perform a marriage for a couple who may already have obtained religious dispensation to marry. They are referred to another state where the jurisdiction permits the marriage of close cousins. This is a case in which the law of the land in about 30 states is more stringent than religious law.

Adult-adult family sexual relationships must be distinguished from adult-child incest because of the legal capacity of the adult to give consent, i.e., mentally competent adults are "equal" and possible consensuality may exist between the participants. Discovery of such incest may be quite accidental. In adult-child cases, whether the child is pre or post-pubertal may be significant in management. If the father is a pedophilic, he will seek a young child of either sex and usually will lose sexual interest after the child becomes physically mature. The father will then be driven by his compulsion to seek another pre-pubertal child (perhaps a younger sibling to the one presenting). The father may consider a natural child merely available and convenient. Coitus may or may not be involved in pedophilia (Maisch, 1972).

Psychosocial

The following classification is proposed to describe all incest cases:
  A. *INCEST DIAGNOSIS*
   1. Consanguineous (blood relative) or affinity (related by marriage)
   2. Consensual, coercive or forceful
   3. Coital or non-coital
   4. Heterosexual or homosexual
   5. Adult-adult, child-child, adult-child, group combination(s)
   6. Rape
   7. Pedophilic
   8. Exhibitionist
   9. Multiple deviance (exploitation, prostitution, transvestism, "kiddie porn," sadomasochism, etc.)
   10. Fantasy/dream
   11. Incest craving/envy
   12. Incest-accepting family/culture/religion
  B. *PHYSICAL DIAGNOSIS* Pregnancy, gonorrhea, vaginal tears, vaginal infection, bruises, or other evidence of assault.
  C. *PSYCHIATRIC DIAGNOSIS* No psychiatric diagnosis, alcohol abuse, drug abuse, mental retardation, depressive disorder, psychosis, conversion disorder, anxiety disorder, dissociative disorder.

Clarity of definition could be of great value in the final understanding and treatment of the "incests" which manifest in clinical practice. The more comprehensive the description, the more helpful. Justification for a separate Category A: "Incest Diagnosis" is that clinically and culturally some incest behaviors are not only accepted but expected and may not be damaging to an individual or the community.

THEORIES OF THE CAUSE OF INCEST

Generally there are alternative courses of action for most human behaviors. In the current context, the question is why some other non-incestuous sexual alternative is not chosen. It may be helpful in management to ask the participants if they can think of sexual alternatives to incest, and why other reasonable possibilities were excluded and incest chosen.

"Opportunity" is often given as an answer, but is not sufficient in itself, as a condition for incest. Others have similar opportunity but choose adultery. In most instances where there is ample opportunity incest does not occur. Poverty and overcrowded living conditions may, but do not always, promote incest. What might the differences be between occurrence and nonoccurrence of incest in situations where opportunities exist?

Personality Profile

Is there a personality profile that predisposes toward incest? Factors that have been theorized include social isolation, lowered inhibitions, alcohol and drug abuse, and psychosis (Weinberg, 1955). Also important is ignorance of appropriate sexual and family relationships (Renshaw, 1981).

Social isolation can and often does exist in crowded urban settings. An individual's capacity to make personal relationships inside and outside the family must then be evaluated. Lowered inhibitory control of sex impulses has been suggested as another contributing personality factor. Heavy alcohol consumption has frequently been mentioned, though in taking case histories it is often difficult to distinguish whether alcohol is a causal factor, contrived excuse, or a rationalization (Virkkunen, 1974).

Incest is *not* only a blue collar phenomenon. It occurs in families of ministers or physicians or wealthy and educated groups. In many instances, when impelling forces are stronger, an incestuous relationship develops despite strong learned sexual inhibitions. One possible condition lowering controls is psychosis, but even the non-psychotic individual may struggle with an overriding incestuous need or fantasy accompanied by strong conflicting feelings which present their own set of management problems.

Inadequate sex education or ignorance regarding the illegality of incest may be a contributory factor in some instances. While greater sexual knowledge and understanding are an important part of individual development, it is unknown whether better sex education could be sufficient to prevent incest in the face of strong predisposing forces. People frequently drink alcohol to excess, chain-smoke cigarettes, and abuse drugs despite an awareness that harmful personal and legal consequences may result. Emotional need often overcomes reason, even when the behavior is known to be self-destructive. This may be true also in cases of incest. Understanding the very close relationship between a need for affectionate touching and the possibility that sustained touching can proceed to sexual arousal (in either or both participants) is an important awareness. This knowledge is crucial for every protective parent, whose task it is to prevent the inappropriate sexualization of affection within the family. Parents must also teach the right to privacy of the body and develop good communication with each child, so that even sexual matters may be discussed. It is also worth mentioning that any "secret" creates some anxiety and a sensitive parent will understand a child's dilemma at needing to confide about incest yet fearing the consequences of "telling."

TREATMENT OF INCEST

In some situations incest is merely noted, recorded, or observed by the anthropologist, sociologist, or researcher with no intervention required.

It is crucial that scholars, professionals in the legal system, and clinicians all be aware of their personal reactions and attitudes toward the very complex problem of incest. Attitudes are always a blend of beliefs and emotions and influence everyday behavior both personal and professional. Expectable normal "entry anxiety" about (1) unknowns and (2) personal competence will surface in the early phases of dealing with incest. Skill, confidence, and comfort result from knowledge and actual practice. A noncondemning acceptance of the participants (the person(s), not necessarily of their behavior) and of the family is an important part of treatment.

Phase One

The first phase of treatment is usually handled by the family physician in a crisis of pregnancy, incestuous rape, or referral to check for child abuse. Usually a minor is involved. The task has medical, legal, and psychological components, and may be tense and time-consuming, often involving more than one discipline.

Data gathering in explicit detail is an essential step in management of incest. There may be many family members to be questioned. One valuable aid is an Incest History Sheet devised in 1979 at the Loyola University of Chicago Department of Psychiatry (Table 1). The structure provided by the explicit History Sheet has been valuable in anxiety reduction, both in the interviewer and in the patient, since its very existence reduces the overwhelming sense of uniqueness and isolation. The History Sheet may be self-administered; however the development of a therapeutic relationship is better served by its face-to-face use, to observe the emotions evoked by the information shared.

When needed, physical examination must proceed with every effort to

TABLE 1. INCEST HISTORY SHEET

	Never		Sometimes		Frequently	
Fantasy only						
Breast/genital fondling						
Deep kissing						
Masturbation of you						
Masturbation by you of kin						
Oral-genital contact						
Anal contact						
Intercourse						
Climax: (a) you (b) kin	(a)	(b)	(a)	(b)	(a)	(b)
Pregnancy						
Fear						
Pain						
Force						
Shame or guilt						
Thoughts about incest						
Dreams about incest						
Reporting to another						
Police/hospital						

	Good	Average	Poor
Relationship between mother and father			
Sex relationship between mother and father			
Relationship between mother and self (a) past (b) now			
Relationship between father and self (a) past (b) now			
Relationship of incest partner and self (a) past (b) now			
Relationship with teacher			
Relationship with minister			
Relationship with spouse now			

allay the anxiety of a child, teen, or adult about (1) being in a hospital or a doctor's office, (2) being questioned, (3) separation from parent(s) or home, (4) fear of pain, (5) fear of harm to family, (6) real pain, (7) other. Dignity may be acknowledged by: the presence of a nurse chaperone, use of adequate body cover (e.g. a sheet), even during necessary genital/rectal exams, use of a tiny nasal speculum for a child's vaginal exam and explaining to the child every step of the way what is being done and why.

If there has been real physical harm or coercion, the physician's task is to recognize child abuse and to protect the minor by involving a Child

Kinship of person who made sex overtures: _____

Was he/she drinking at the time? _____ Threat? _____ Violence? _____

Did he/she have (a) sex with other family members? ____ (b) Psychiatric problem(s)? ____

Your age at time: _____ Kin's age at time: _____

How did it end? _____

Did you like this person? _____

Do you see each other now? _____ Details: _____

_____

Person told to keep it secret? _____ Feelings about the secret? _____

Did you tell? _____ Details: _____

Did someone else tell? _____

Details: _____

Pregnancy (if any): _____ Outcome: _____ VD Yes/No Outcome: _____

Preoccupations with incest (present)? _____

Preoccupations with incest (past)? _____

Dreams about incest (present)? _____

Dreams about incest (past)? _____

Reading about incest (past): _____ Present: _____

Does your spouse know about this? _____

Reaction: _____

Need for Psychotherapy (past): _____ Present: _____

Sex problems in past: _____

Sex problems now: _____

Details: _____

What helped you most to handle or resolve your feelings about the incest? _____

_____

Protection Agency. To do this there must be reasonable physician certainty that the incest charge is neither a hoax nor a malicious accusation, both of which have occurred, although rarely, and may have destructive repercussions for all involved. A Child Advocacy Team or a Hospital Rape Team may be of some help with time-consuming legal contacts. Court hearings may involve more time at a later date. Records must be precise and complete since they will be later requested by the courts. Publicity and court hearings may be very traumatic for the whole family, who could benefit from sensitive supportive professional help.

Phase Two

The second phase of treatment usually involves a psychiatric evaluation of the incest participant(s) often upon order of the court in cases of child-adult cases, but only occasionally for adult-adult incest. These may be either coital or non-coital.

After careful data gathering and an explicit incest history (Table 1), the court deliberations will proceed upon the psychiatrist's psychodynamic formulation of this case. Since incest occurs in a family context, as many family members as possible should be seen to complete the picture and describe the context within which the incest took place.

Is this family from an incest-accepting culture? Is it a natural, divorced, or reconstituted family? What is the sexual adjustment of the parent couple? (This is the essential nurturant dyad: if there is a fulfilling exchange emotionally and sexually, why turn to a child?) Is there a psychiatric or police history: pedophilia, exhibitionism, manic depression, alcoholism, or drug abuse? What about protection of a minor by the other parent? And the relationships with other family members and the extended family network?

From all of this and more, the psychodynamic formulation must be woven for the courts to assist understanding of this particular family. Then the diagnosis must be made: (1) Incest Diagnosis, (2) Physical Diagnosis, (3) Psychiatric Diagnosis, as already outlined.

Prognosis and Management Recommendations must also be made for the minor (if any), for the adult participant(s), for the family, and for follow-up.

One should recognize that in cases of incest, legal and social intervention by the courts and other public agencies, when inappropriate and insensitive, can compound what may already be a serious problem. Self-righteous condemnation and a punitive attitude, although well-meaning, may lead to destruction of the family unit and institutionalization of some of the parties involved. This may well be more traumatic than the initial incest. Prolonged "over-questioning" of participants may turn into humiliating inquisition. Privacy is a precious human right to be honored and invaded only with respect.

In incest situations, the program must be aimed at treatment of the problems of those who present and *not* the emotions triggered in the personnel who are directing the interview. Moral outrage on the part of a professional may have particularly destructive clinical consequences. Note the particular problems each incest participant and family has, since it is impossible to make general rules to serve the best interests of all persons. There may be times when the best approach in dealing with the problem is to remove one or more individuals from the family, but often removal may jeopardize the possible benefits of intensive family therapy in an intact family unit.

For child-adult incest, whether non-coital, non-coercive, affinity, or otherwise, the primary consideration is whether there can be assurance, with professional intervention, of child protection. If so, after legal preliminaries and with possible court order, the difficult first goal of treatment is to engage the bruised family in therapy and build a relationship of trust with the therapist. This will take time and testing. It is also essential to build trust *within* the family relationships—between parents, between parent and the child incest participants, between siblings. No matter what the illusions may be, there are few secrets in a family; "everyone knows but nobody says." Treatment will be a long and sometimes stormy course, but slowly centers doing good work with incest cases are emerging providing data that support therapeutic optimism. (Giarretto et al., 1978; Renshaw, 1977).

CONCLUSION

Incest taboos have shaped human society since the beginning of recorded history. Incest has been considered by some sociologists to be the most extreme form of deviant behavior—the "universal crime"—yet it is also behavior noted in nearly all cultures, some of which accept and mandate its practice. Psychosexual development occurs—for better or for worse—within the intimacy of family life, which may include crowded quarters, common beds, relaxation of dress codes, exposure to nudity, and a total absence of sex education. Sexual arousal feelings are undifferentiated and may be elicited in the adult by a child and vice-versa. Such feelings must be acknowledged, understood, and controlled as part of maturation and gradual learning. It may well evolve that failure to desexualize affectionate family closeness can be considered a sexual learning defect. This will take on special significance in cases of affinity (post-divorce or other newly constituted families), in which protective desexualization of affection has not had time to develop.

The severity of coercion, timing, repetition, gentleness, or important closeness of the incestuous act are all features which will mark the ultimate personal outcome as positive or negative. Some persons will integrate the experience, gain perspective, and exhibit no distress or problems. Others may feel severe discomfort when mere thoughts of incest intrude. Each deserve careful, open-minded evaluation.

Much remains to be understood about incest. Further study is hampered by current criminalization of incest and global categorization of "any" sex act between adult and child as child abuse, reportable by law. Special privilege laws favor doctor-patient confidentiality and may be exercised. These laws do not extend to other health care professionals, who may report to the law before evaluation is complete and lose the family to treatment by provoking actual flight from their home and state. Adequate study may only proceed if decriminalization occurs. Current understanding and treatment of incest *cannot* be regarded as satisfactory. Better knowledge of the problem, including why it does *not* occur in some families, can provide tools to identify incest cases and lead to prevention through adequate education for individuals, the family, and the community.

REFERENCES

Cohen Y: The disappearance of the incest taboo. *Hum Nature:* 72–76, July 1978

Ford CS, Beach FA: *Patterns of Sexual Behavior.* New York, Harper & Row Publishers, Inc., 1970

Giarretto H, Giarretto A, Sgroi S: Coordinated community treatment of incest, in Burgess AW et al: *Sexual Assault of Children and Adolescents.* Lexington, Mass, Lexington Books, 1978, pp. 231–240

Maisch H: *Incest,* Bearne C (trans). New York, Stein and Day, 1972

Renshaw DC: Healing the incest wound. *Sex Med Today* 1 (1):27–41, October 1977

Renshaw DC: *Incest—Understanding and Treatment.* Boston, Little, Brown & Co. 1981

Renshaw DC, Renshaw RH: Incest. *J Sex Educ Therapy* 3:2 (winter): 3–7, 1977

Virkkunen M: Incest offenses and alcoholism. *Med Sci Law* 14: 124–128, April 1974

Weinberg SK: *Incest.* New York, Citadel, 1955

2

Sadomasochism

Jon K. Meyer and Carol Dupkin

Sadism and masochism are often considered purely in a sexual context. However, sadistic or masochistic practices serve a larger function. Sadomasochism is universal in perversion, where it *is* eroticized, and in transsexualism, where it *is not*.

In both perversion and transsexualism, sadomasochism is an expression of aggression. As such, it has the function of defining and controlling a particular version of reality which arbitrates the anatomical differences between the sexes, the continuum between individuation and merger, and the balance sheet of narcissistic supplies. We believe that a critical phase in defining these realities—and, therefore, a critical phase in the pathology of perversion and transsexualism—is the period of pre-oedipal genital interest at age 18 months.

In developing our thesis we will touch on the similarities, distinctions, and relationships between perversion and gender disorder, the function of the drives and drive discharge in the affirmation of the self and reality, the narcissistic economy in perversion and gender disorder, and the role of object relations in self/non-self and sexual distinctions.

THE MOTIVE FORCE: LIBIDINAL AND AGGRESSIVE DRIVES

With the ascendance of the structural model, ego psychology, and object relations theory, the eminence of drive psychology has faded. Nonetheless, in the study of patients with sadomasochistic and transsexual proclivities, one is clearly reminded of the existence of the drives.

While sexuality has, over the years, lost its special theoretical role in development it is still the most archaic mode, closely tied to the primary process, and for that reason especially capable of expressing the emotional truth of personal existence. Furthermore, with the development of orgastic capacity, the sexual drive acquires a powerful mode of full discharge, which serves as an adjunct for the affirmation of identity and personal reality. Orgasm has been called a "triumph of realization which for an instant gives eminent life and power to the thoughts that surge on its crest" (Nydes, 1950). Eissler (1958) has credited orgasm with the power to confirm, create, and affirm beliefs, providing the individual with a conviction of the truthfulness and reality of the images he is consciously or unconsciously entertaining at the moment of climax. Stolorow has suggested that orgasm in perversion serves to restore the structurally-deficient person's conviction of having a bounded and cohesive self.

The constraints of libidinal and aggressive drives are different. The full, unsublimated discharge of sexual drives in intercourse and orgasm does no harm to the participants. Unsublimated aggressive discharge is literally destructive. The fact that libidinal drives have a ready outlet, while the aggressive drives do not, probably accounts for the frequent aggressive (sadistic or masochistic) contamination of sexuality. In addition to the borrowed sexual avenue, aggression finds a more or less sublimated outlet in the processes of definition and control. If libidinal trends are colored by fusion, merger, attachment, and love, aggression is characterized by discrimination, declaration, and assertion. Bach and Schwartz (1972) have noted that the function of affirmation may also be served by fantasies of revenge and sacrifice. In this regard, the aggression in masochism and sadism functions narcissistically to restore and maintain cohesiveness, stability, and affect balance.

Control is an essential ingredient in symptomatology. The symptom or character deformation is a compromise among the forces serving to control inner and outer pressures. In the area of the mind where a pathological formation holds sway, time is frozen in place, anatomical reality may be negated or falsified, and childhood traumata with their childhood solutions are endlessly replayed. The crystallized center of the pathological formation expresses the reality within which identity is defined. Perversion and gender disorder have in common not only the peculiar libidinal attachments, but also the essential and brittle control exercised over object-representations. This control is central in the patient's narcissistic economy.

While in perversion, particularly sadomasochistic perversion, the blending of sexuality and aggression serves many purposes, the aspect we wish to emphasize is that of assertion. In perversion, orgasm is involved, not so much as an end in itself, but as an adjunct to the ratification of a particular self-concept and view of reality. Pain and dominance in sexuality, either enforced actively or experienced passively, define the boundaries of the self. In transsexuality, the developmentally more advanced function of orgasm is often abandoned. Reality and self are structured by maternal fusion—a more primitive aspect of sexuality—and by genital ablation and sterilization, which are unquestionably more primitive aspects of aggression.

OBJECTS AND STRUCTURE

Relationships among members of the nuclear family contribute to the form and substance of perversion and gender pathology (Meyer, 1980a, 1980b, in press; Meyer and Dupkin, in press). Libidinal and aggressive undercurrents are communicated in handling, feeding, cleaning, and training children. In the family which may generate perversion or gender disorder there is uneasiness at both intimacy and separation, magical investment in talisman objects, tacit enactment of prohibitions and seductions, and strongly held mythology about the differences between the sexes, procreation, and birth. Children form emotional resonances to their family's unspoken wishes and unconscious needs, profoundly affecting their sense of self.

A fundamental task of early development is the child's gradual "separation" and "individuation" from the mother (Mahler et al., 1975). Mother constitutes not only a major element of the neonate's physical environment, but also the emotional universe in which he is imbedded. The change from neonate to toddler to first grader involves not only physical maturation but also emotional enfranchisement.

One of the earliest discriminations in the developing sense of self is the distinction between "me" and "not me," beginning at around four or five months of age. A second major discrimination is the recognition of the anatomical distinctions between the sexes at approximately 18 months. This latter distinction is established roughly between the practicing and the rapprochement subphases of separation-individuation, is closely associated with the anal phase and toileting, and is contemporaneous with the period of gender formation. That second major discrimination, and its context, seems pivotal in the production of gender disorder and perversion. What occurs at this crucial pass is not only cognitive recognition of male-female differences, but also a readjustment of emotional reality. The real distinctions in sexual anatomy seem to confront the vulnerable child with a perplexing and disturbing discontinuity.

Galenson, Roiphe, and their associates have investigated the period of 18-month genital interest. This early genital phase occurs coincidentally with what is known, from independent sources, as the critical phase for gender development (Hampson and Hampson, 1961; Money et al., 1955a, 1955b, 1956). Their observations suggest that this pre-oedipal genital orientation is part of a process of object and self-consolidation and body-genital schematization. Severe reactions to discovery of sexual differences have been noted in certain children, and these reactions seemed to be associated with anxieties of object and self-annihilation. In the course of these reactions the children have manifested "fetishistic" attachments to inanimate objects and "sadomasochistic" relationships with parents and siblings (Roiphe, 1968; Roiphe and Galenson, 1972, 1973; Galenson and Roiphe, 1971; Galenson et al., 1975).

The process of integrating sexual distinctions appears particularly difficult for the infant whose mother suffers from excessive separation anxiety, anal fixations, penis envy, and phallic preoccupations (Lihn, 1971). Her difficulties tend to be expressed through control over the child and his bodily functions. The child experiences being possessed and penetrated, alternating with being rejected and disregarded. Attempts are made to relieve the separation anxiety by creating substitutes for the mother-child union, often through a peculiar autoeroticism, utilizing bodily parts and objects linked to both mother and child. In this process, the distinctions between the sexes are blurred. Unfortunately, a solid hold on the anatomical distinctions between sexes is an essential component of developing body image. Without that hold, the glue of an emotionally solid, stable body image does not set and body parts are perceived as though in constant danger of coming apart. Appendages are imbued with more aggression than usual. The maturing sexual drives are distorted in the interest of bolstering body image, lending sexual relationships more narcissistic than object-related value (Greenacre, 1968; Goldberg, 1975). As the early relationship with mother is peculiar, and lacking in the uncomplicated qualities of "freely enough given" empathy and affection, a wish develops to compel through force what is not given out of love. In this way aggressive drives are exaggerated in the service of narcissistic needs. Given an unstable body image, an identification with mother, anxious body narcissism, and an exaggeration of aggressive drives, it is easy to imagine the state of vulnerability in the 18-month crisis. Under such circumstances, merger, fusion, control, and self-sacrifice replace progressive development.

SADISM AND MASOCHISM

In sadism and masochism, issues of control, domination, subjugation, and aggression are clearly and overtly enacted. In sexual masochism, excitement is linked with the passive experience of physical or emotional subjugation (which may be simulated or real). Sexual sadism is the direct reciprocal, in which excitement is linked to the active infliction (in fantasy or reality) of danger, humiliation, subjugation, abuse, or torture. Sadism and masochism, respectively, are active and passive representatives of aggressive control functions. Although relatively pure sadists or masochists exist, most commonly the active or passive perversion is preferential but not absolute. Sadists also indulge in masochistic fantasies or practices, and the subjugated, compliant masochist is often quite able to take the opposite role with arousal and pleasure.

One of the aspects of the self-representation which is pathologically defined through the masochist's suffering or the sadist's power is gender identity. In perversion, gender sense is preserved and defined by aggression, both actual and symbolic, in the sadomasochistic ritual. The use of sacrifice, pain, and mutilation to define the boundaries of the self, to secure gender sense, and to freeze psychic reality, however, is not limited to its symbolic use in the perversions. Pursuit of similar goals, but with an abandonment of orgasm and a partial breakdown of the symbolization process, occurs in transsexualism. The transsexual's request for sex reassignment, for what may serve as a controlled "mutilation," can be understood as a sadomasochistic process in which symbolization has failed.

PERVERSION AND GENDER DISORDER: THE CLINICAL PICTURE

The richness in perversion gives rise to a welter of clinical descriptors, e.g., voyeurism, homosexuality, transvestism, sadism, and masochism. These clinical descriptors do not define entities, but rather indicate variations on a common theme. These varieties are distinguished by specialized sexual fantasies, masturbatory practices, sexual props, and expectations of the sexual partner, but the manifest perverse symptom is only the most conspicuous part of an underlying sadomasochistic character structure (Lihn, 1971).

Paralleling the scope of symptomatology, there is a spectrum in perverse psychopathology. At one end, perversion shades into the psychoses and gender identity disorders, while at the other, perversity gradually becomes repressed in the neuroses (Meyer, 1980b). In other words, the range of ego strengths is enormous, a fact which gives rise to emphasis on both the centrality of the castration complex (Bak, 1968) and the importance of pre-oedipal factors (Greenacre, 1953, 1955, 1960). Nevertheless, it is generally acknowledged among those who stress phallic-oedipal factors that pre-oedipal disturbances are their forerunners. As Bak (1968) noted, patients with sadomasochistic perversions had intense dyadic relationships with much physical closeness and associated sensitivity to separation.

The themes and variations of perversion extend into the gender identity disorders and are reflected in transsexual syndromes with admixtures of homosexuality, transvestism, polymorphous perversity, etc. (Meyer, 1974). At their core, however, the apparently diverse conditions have common features.

The transsexual's conscious endorsement of the cross-sexual wish is the focal point of the syndrome and the organizing motif of his life. The quest for sex reassignment has, as its essence, a sense of disconnection between anatomy and self-representation. There is a clear awareness of physiognomy but a disavowal of its significance. It seems clear that such disconnection and disavowal are accomplished only at the price of a split in the ego (Freud, 1940a). The ego modifications in transsexualism are a split in relation to anatomy with denial of the relevance of anatomical givens, acceptance and endorsement of genital ablation, and the devotion of the ego's executive apparatus to symptomatic wish fulfillment (Meyer, in press). Ubiquitous sadistic and masochistic elements in transsexualism sometimes appear to be institutionalized in the relationship with "gender" programs which embody the potential or actual surgical sacrifice of genitalia and reproductive organs. This relationship *is not* overtly eroticized and is not directed toward orgastic discharge. It *is* devoted to issues of self-definition, control, and reparation.

Stoller (1975) has viewed transsexualism as an identity *per se* rather than as a symptomatic attempt to preserve a threatened and fragile identity. In Stoller's frame of reference, a distinction *in kind* rather than *of degree* is made between perversion and transsexualism. Our experience in providing psychiatric services to transsexual patients over the past ten years has led us to the opposite conclusion: namely, that transsexualism is *of a kind* with perversion. The cross-sexual identifications in perversion are universal and often obvious but the wishes for gender transmutation, while sometimes conscious, do not emerge with any power unless perverse defenses fail (Bak, 1968). The symbolic control exercised through paraphilic fantasies and rituals maintains the repression of gender-fragmenting impulses and cross-sexual wishes. In the transsexual, symbolization has failed and what is contained by fantasy in perversion must be made concrete in transsexualism.

It seems to us that transsexualism and perversion both stand astride the 18-month critical phase, but look in different directions: perversion looks ahead to object-constancy and the sexuality of the phallic-oedipal phase; transsexualism looks backward to global identification and merger. The following case may help to illustrate this point.

A young man in late adolescence was brought for consultations by his parents because of his apparently ardent desire for reassignment surgery. His father, who had suffered from a paranoid psychosis and alcoholism, had been intimately and seductively involved in his sons's upbringing. The mother, who was depressive, had never separated from her family and was tied to her depressed mother and alcoholic father by strong and ambivalent bonds. The patient's family supported his pursuit of surgery, stating that they were willing to do anything that might make their son happy. The patient was, indeed, an unhappy young man. In early adolescence he had gone through a painful time of "not knowing who or what I was" that culminated in a suicide attempt. He had emerged from the attempted suicide with a conviction of really being a girl and a resolve to pursue surgery.

At the time the patient was first seen he reported not being able to ejaculate under any circumstances. He had no sexual fantasies and no erotic dreams. An attempt was made to dissuade him from pursuing surgery and psychotherapy was recommended.

The patient was seen again two years later. At that time he was a bearded, leather-jacketed, effeminate homosexual, who had discovered that he could ejaculate after being beaten by a man. The ejaculation was accompanied by a fantasy of going into the basement with his father, being beaten by him, and emerging from the cellar with a sense of ecstatic union despite the pain. For the moment, at least, his quest for sex reassignment was abandoned.

What had been concrete in the search for sex reassignment became symbolic in the perversion and was controlled by fantasy and displacement. The symbolization, however, was of a primitive sort utilizing a primary object. Discovery of a means to have orgasm engendered a progressive developmental push and was associated with a modicum of symbolic control over female identification and masochistic sacrifice.

CONCLUSION

The paraphilias are a large and significant group of disorders with intrinsic core fantasies, sexual scripts, stagings, supporting players, props, and audiences. The core fantasy contains the kernel of condensed, steadfast childhood beliefs.

We would postulate that the essential features of perversion are a blurring of sexual and generational differences and a poor infant-mother demarcation, particularly in the realm of the genitalia. There is impairment of gender and reality senses. The paraphilia serve to symbolically cover flaws in the perception of bodily integrity and reality. Sadomasochistic processes in perversion control traumatic reality and maintain narcissistic balance. Despite the severity of the fantasies (even in sadomasochism), perversion is a fundamentally progressive symptom in which physical integrity is protected.

The essential features in transsexualism are similar blurring of sexual and generational differences and poor separation between the representations of self and mother. The impairment of reality sense is more conspicuous than in perversion, with the denial of the meaning of anatomical givens approaching psychotic concreteness. The possibility of symbolic control is abandoned and the sacrifice of genitalia enacts, matter-of-factly, the ultimate masochistic sacrifice.

From the perspective of the 18-month critical phase of body-genital schematization, perversion embodies progressive trends with the incorporation of orgasm and phallic investment in an attempt to maintain a hold on phallic-oedipal organization. Transsexualism, as it were, looks backward. Symbolization and orgasm, as progressive trends, cannot be sustained. Global identity and fusion, which are necessary to defend against the threat of disintegration and annihilation, are achieved through masochistic sacrifice. This sacrifice, however, is a narcissistic triumph of megalomaniacal proportions.

REFERENCES

Bach S, Schwartz L: A dream of the Marquis de Sade. *J Am Psychoanal Assoc* 20:451–475, 1972

Bak R: The phallic woman: the ubiquitous fantasy in perversion. *Psychoanal Study Child* 23:15–36, 1968

Eissler K: Notes on problems of technique in the psychoanalytic treatment of adolescents: With some remarks on perversion. *Psychoanal Study Child* 13:223–254, 1958

Freud S: Three essays on the theory of sexuality. *Standard Edition.* 23(7):125–243, 1905

Freud S: The splitting of the ego in the process of defense. *Standard Edition* 23:273–278, 1940a

Freud S: An outline of psychoanalysis. *Standard Edition* 23:141–207, 1940b

Galenson E, Roiphe H: The impact of early sexual discovery on mood, defensive organization and symbolization. *Psychoanal Study Child* 26:195–216, 1971

Galenson E, Roiphe H: Some suggested revisions concerning early female development. *J Am Psychoanal Assoc* 24(5):29–57, 1976

Galenson E, Vogel S, Blau S, Roiphe H: Disturbance in sexual identity beginning at 18 months of age. *Int Rev Psychoanal* 2:389–397, 1975

Goldberg D: A fresh look at perverse behavior. *Int J Psychoanal* 56:335–342, 1975

Greenacre P: Certain relationships between fetishism and faculty development of the body image. *Psychoanal Study Child* 8:79–98, 1953

Greenacre P: Further considerations regarding fetishism. *Psychoanal Study Child* 10:187–194, 1955

Greenacre P: Further notes on fetishism. *Psychoanal Study Child* 15:191–207, 1960

Greenacre P: Perversions: General considerations regarding their genetic and dynamic background. *Psychoanal Study Child* 23:47–62, 1968

Hampson JL, Hampson JG: The ontogenesis of sexual behavior in man, in Young W (ed): *Sex and Internal Secretions,* vol 2. Baltimore, Williams and Wilkins, 1961 pp 1401–1432

Lichtenstein J: Identity and sexuality: A study of their interrelationships in man. *J Am Psychoanal Assoc* 9:197–260, 1961

Lihn H: Sexual masochism: A case report. *Int J Psychoanal* 52:469–478, 1971

Mahler K, Pine F, Bergman A: *The Psychological Birth of the Human Infant.* New York, Basic Books, 1975

Meyer J: Clinical variants among applicants for sex reassignment. *Arch Sex Behav* 3:527–558, 1974

Meyer J: Body image, selfness, and gender sense. *Psych Clinics North America,* 3:21–36, 1980a

Meyer J: Paraphilia, in Kaplan H, Freedman A, Sadock E (eds): *Comprehensive*

Textbook of Psychiatry, ed 3. Baltimore, Williams and Wilkins, 1980b, pp 1770–1782

Meyer J: The theory of the gender identity disorders. *J am Psychoanal Assoc,* in press

Meyer J, Dupkin C: Environment and gender identity, in Gilmore D, Cook B (eds): *Environmental Factors in Mammalian Reproduction.* London, Macmillan, in press

Money J, Hampson JG, Hampson JL: Hermaphroditism: Recommendations concerning assignment of sex, change of sex, and psychologic management. *Bull JHH* 97:284–300, 1955a

Money J, Hampson JG, Hampson JL: An examination of some basic sexual concepts: The evidence of human hermaphroditism. *Bull JHH* 97:301–319, 1955b

Money J, Hampson JG, Hampson JL: Sexual incongruities and psychopathology: The evidence of human hermaphroditism. *Bull JHH* 98:43–57, 1956

Nydes J: The magical experience of the masturbation fantasy. *Am J Psychother* 4:303–310, 1950

Roiphe H: On an early genital phase with an addendum on genesis. *Psychoanal Study Child* 23:348–365, 1968

Roiphe H, Galenson E: Early genital activity and the castration complex. *Psychoanal Q* 41:334–347, 1972

Roiphe H, Galenson E: The infantile fetish. *Psychoanal Study Child* 28:147–166, 1973

Stoller R: *Sex and Gender, vol 2: The Transsexual Experiment.* New York, Aronson, 1975

Stolorow R: Addendum to a partial analysis of a perversion involving bugs: An illustration of the narcissistic function of perverse activity. *Int J Psychoanal* 56:361–364, 1975

Stolorow R: The narcissistic function of masochism (and sadism). *Int J Psychoanal* 56:441–448, 1975b

3

Rape

Richard T. Rada

INTRODUCTION

Violent behavior has reached epidemic proportions in America. Each year the FBI Uniform Crime Reports indicate a steady increase in violent crimes such as rape, murder, and assault and battery. It is almost axiomatic that when society's experts in common sense become baffled by a problem, society turns to its experts in uncommon sense for understanding and solution. Historically, however, mental health professional interest in violent behaviors such as rape has been sporadic; professional involvement has been characterized by short-term bursts of activity often prompted by sensational newspaper headlines about an unusually bizarre or repulsive offense. Sustained long-term commitment to understanding basic causes and motivations for such acts has been lacking.

In recent years, the women's movement has been responsible in large measure for a more persistent focus on crimes of sexual abuse and assault. As a result, the too long neglected areas of victim response and victim care are now being actively studied. Concomitantly, a number of investigators have begun to examine the biological, psychological, and sociological factors prompting rapists' behavior. Although the psychology of the rapist remains poorly understood, there is growing consensus regarding certain facets of rapists' behavior. The purpose of this presentation is to examine the psychological motivation of the rapist, to highlight recent concern about rape of male victims by male offenders, and to discuss possible prevention strategies.

PSYCHOLOGICAL MOTIVATION OF THE RAPIST

Professionals who have studied rapists firsthand are initially impressed by the variety of myths that have arisen over the years regarding rapists and rape offenses (Rada, 1977; Groth and Birnbaum, 1979). Although professional disagreements about certain aspects of rapists' behavior exist, there now appears to be general agreement about the following four points:

1. There is no such thing as a typical rapist in regard to personality type or motivation.

2. Rape is an act which combines aggressive and sexual elements; the degree and manner in which these two psychological factors are combined in and expressed by the individual rapist do vary.

3. With rare exception, rape does not appear to be prompted by the absence of voluntary sexual partners.

4. In the vast majority of cases, rape is not an impulsive act prompted by a spur of the moment sexual or aggressive feeling, but is rather a planned act, often designed in a meticulous manner.

Historically, rape has been viewed at various times as a mainly sexual act; recently, rape has more often been described as primarily an aggressive act. Several factors, however, mitigate against viewing rape as either pure aggression or pure sexuality. Identification of sexual desire as the sole motivation for rape does not account for the fact that many rapists are married at the time of the commission of the offense and that many others admit to being involved in satisfactory voluntary sexual relationships with women friends during the period when they are also engaged in rape. If rape were motivated solely by aggression and hostility, it would make sense that such desires would be more simply satisfied by physically assaulting the victim.

Rape is a crime that combines both sexual and aggressive components. Feelings of aggression and sexuality are common to all of us but only a few men rape. What then has gone awry in the melding of these emotions in the rapist that prompts him to commit an act that causes so much physical and psychic distress?

An obvious first question is whether rapists differ from "normals" in regard to their hostility and sexuality. Unfortunately, the literature on hostility of the rapist is scanty. Our group has conducted several studies measuring scores of rapists on various self-report psychometric tests that purport to measure both the trait and state of hostility (Rada et al., 1976; Rada et al., unpublished). Rapists do score higher on hostility rating scales in these studies than normals or child molesters, a group considered to be nonviolent. Several methodologic problems with these studies, however, confound the conclusions to be drawn from the data. First, the studies are based on convicted rapists, a fact that immediately introduces a sampling bias. Second, the mean group scores of rapists are higher, but there are many individual rapists who score at or below the level of normals. Third, the validity of hostility rating scales and the construct they purport to measure are subject to question (Buss et al., 1962). Moreover, a substantial minority of convicted rapists display sociopathic personality disorders, and can be expected to have a history of more frequent antisocial and aggressive acts besides rape. No other studies have systematically examined the trait or state of hostility in rapists.

Analysis of rapists' marital relationships might provide some insight into rapists' general level of hostility, but the reports in the literature are conflicting. Glueck is cited as saying that the hostility of sex offenders toward women is so great that it precludes a happy, stable marriage (Shultz, 1965). On the other hand, individual case histories and direct reports from rapists themselves indicate that some rapists have relatively stable or satisfactory marriages (Karpman, 1950; Wille, 1961). Although some are physically assaultive with their wives—in our experience, sociopathic or sociopathic alcoholic types (Rada, 1978), most do not appear to be sexually aggressive. This may explain why wives of rapists are frequently surprised when informed of their husbands' rape activity.

Given that rape is an aggressive offense, the amount of violence used by rapists in committing the offense can be viewed on a continuum from the most brutal rapist to the least violent rapist who uses only verbal threats and subsequently commits the sexual intercourse without inflicting physical injury on the victim. Viewed in this manner, only a minority of convicted rapists commit the most violent type of offense.

In summary, there is some data that rapists as a group evidence more hostility than non-rapists, but the data is meager; when rapists are considered individually there is marked variation in hostility scores.

Sexuality of the Rapist

For many reasons, data on the strength of sex offenders' sexual drive remains anecdotal, based primarily on individual case reports. From a theoretical viewpoint, sexual paraphilias and sex offenses have been considered the result of lack of control in "oversexed" persons or, conversely, as compensatory behavior in individuals who are "undersexed."

There is little objective evidence for either view. Moreover, such notions are confounded by the fact that the frequency and adequacy of sexual response among "normals" is highly variable and difficult to estimate.

Sexual dysfunction in the history of sex offenders has been studied. Glueck (1956) found that thirteen percent of rapists reported a history of episodic or chronic severe disturbance in sexual performance. Gebhard et al. (1965) did not find a high percentage of impotence among rapists; in my clinical experience, few rapists report persistent chronic difficulties with sexual performance. Impotence or difficulty with ejaculation during the act of rape has been reported in some rapists (Groth and Burgess, 1977). But here again, considering the circumstances under which most rapes occur, and that many rapists have been drinking heavily before the rape, such dysfunction, usually temporary, would not be altogether unexpected. The fact that there is relatively little dysfunction may be the striking finding.

Sadism in the narrow sense of sexual delight in the infliction of physical pain does not appear to be a common feature among rapists. Some rapists are sadistic with their voluntary sex partners as well as during the rape. Infliction of physical pain, however, is not a major motivation of most rapists during rape, and it is rarely the preferred or exclusive form of sexual pleasure for most of these men. Abel et al. (1977) and Barbaree et al. (1979) have measured the sexual arousal of rapists and non-rapists to verbal descriptions of mutually consenting sex, rape, and violent nonsexual assault. Mutually consenting sex evoked sexual arousal in both groups. Rape evoked comparable arousal in rapists but significantly less arousal in non-rapists. The rapists, however, did not exhibit greater sexual arousal to forced or violent sex compared with consenting sex. Thus, it appears that few rapists require or prefer forced sex or violent nonsexual themes to obtain sexual arousal. Karpman noted that pain in connection with rape is incidental; the primary motive is the overcoming of the victim (1959).

The author has noted a finding in rapists' sexual history which may have some significance. Approximately fifty percent of rapists admit to prior acts of sexual deviation such as "peeping", exhibitionism, and fetishism (Rada, 1978a). This finding, coupled with an admission by some rapists of early adolescent fantasies of aggressive sexual desires, suggests that many are themselves aware of basic difficulties in their early sexual development, a point which I shall again address under prevention strategies.

I turn now to my understanding of the primary motivation for rape. Rape is a crime of control, power, and dominance (Rada, 1978a). The primary motive of the rapist is to control the victim. It is in this sense that the aggressive component is more dominant than the sexual component in the rape offense. In fact, for many rapists the sexual act itself appears to be less important than the ritual of the rape event, which is more often carefully planned than impulsive.

Rape then is the means by which the rapist attempts to control the victim and, by extension, all women. The manner in which the rape is effected, or the mode or style of raping, depends in large measure on the admixture of sexual and aggressive desires within the individual rapist. Thus, the manner of raping can be viewed on a continuum from sexual on one end to aggressive on the other end. Some rapists appear to derive more satisfaction from the sexual interaction in rape, whereas others clearly derive their satisfaction from forcibly overcoming the victim and overpowering her resistance. The sadistic rapist can be viewed as resting in the middle of this continuum, where the sexual and aggressive elements tend to fuse and meld. The sadistic rapist often prefers to express his sadism, not through direct infliction of pain, but rather through humiliation of the victim. This frequently takes the form of forcing the victim to commit certain sexual acts, such as cunnilingus and fellatio, which in this context both the victim and the assailant perceive as degrading.

If control is the rapist's basic motivation, why does he attempt to satisfy this desire through a forced sexual act? The reason is that, in the rapist's mind, a woman's sexual intimacy is her most precious example of personal control. Thus, forcing a woman to submit to sexual intercourse is the most potent manner of depriving her of her sense of personal control. It is the utmost in personal domination. This understanding of the motive for rape may explain why rapists not infrequently admit to less satisfaction from a rape when the victim, seeing that there is no other alternative, submits to the act of rape and goes along with the rapist's demands in order to avoid serious injury. The victim's submission, not synonymous with consent, tends to deprive the rapist of the sense of having taken complete control and having completely dominated the victim.

Finally, the most basic question: What is the source of the rapist's desire for control? Rapists characteristically experience a real or imagined inability to establish a satisfying love relationship with a woman. It is interesting that even rapists who appear to be happily married, at least on a superficial basis, often perceive themselves as unable to establish an emotionally gratifying give-and-take relationship with their wives or any other woman. The rapist, unlike other men who experience this same

absence in their lives, responds with a vain attempt to control by force
what he feels inadequate or unable to obtain on a voluntary basis. It is
not, therefore, simply hostility toward women that motivates the rapist.
He attempts to satisfy a felt need, but the sense of control obtained by
force during the rape is not permanently satisfying. What follows in many
rapists is a vicious cycle. In the absence of a satisfying relationship with a
woman, they often turn again to the temporary gratification achieved
through the rape. By doing so, however, they paradoxically become even
more dependent on the victim, a dependence which only further com-
pounds their sense of lack of control.

One important application of this understanding of the motivation of
the rapist relates to the victim-assailant interaction during the rape. It is
likely that the more successful the rapist is in his desire to obtain control
during the rape, the more the victim will be made to feel helpless and
without control. Such feelings in the victim might easily generalize to
other areas in her life after the rape; this development appears to be
confirmed by those studying victims' responses to rape events (Burgess
and Holmstrom, 1974). In addition, one of the reasons that rape by a
psychotic man is such a frightening experience for the victim is that this
is one instance in which neither the rapist nor the victim is in control of
the events.

Detailed study of the individual rapist indicates that many combinations of motives may initiate a rapist's behavior (Groth and Birnbaum,
1979: Rada, 1978a). Rape is a complex offense prompted by an interplay
of biological, psychological, social, and possibly political factors. Complete understanding of the rapist's behavior requires careful attention to
all these factors and components.

RAPE OF MALE VICTIMS BY MALE OFFENDERS

Male Victim Rape in Society

Rape has been defined traditionally as sexual assault by a male against a
female. About ten years ago, professionals began to note an increase in
reports of sexual assault by males against other males. These assaults
frequently involved rape of a pre-adolescent or early adolescent boy by a
late adolescent or young adult male. These attacks, committed by gangs
or one assailant, were often characterized by excessive use of force and
violence toward the victims. This trend has continued (Kaufman et al.,
1980; Groth and Burgess, 1980). In Albuquerque there are two major

rape victim resource services: the Rape Crisis Center and the Sexual Assault Response Team. At present, approximately eight percent of victims seeking help from the Rape Crisis Center are male; the Sexual Assault Response Team reports that approximately ten percent of their victims are male. The age of victims ranges from 5–45 years. Most appear to be stranger rapes, and the victims and the assailant are likely to be of the same race. Victims are generally younger than assailants. Most of these rapes are committed by a rapist acting alone, but a higher percentage of male victims than female victims are attacked by multiple assailants. It is believed, as is the case with female victims, that a large number of rapes of males are unreported.

I have recently become aware of a number of rapes of young male children by adolescent male babysitters. Sexual interaction, voluntary or forced, among babysitters and their charges is not new. The use of male babysitters, however, seems to be increasing and a potential unfortunate and inadvertent consequence may be increased victimization of young children. Such assaults can have serious emotional consequences for the victim, the parents of the victim, and the parents of the assailant. When a male babysitter has seduced or forced sexual activity on a young child, the child is frequently threatened with physical harm if he informs. In such a situation, the child may acquiesce to further sexual assault rather than risk the imagined greater danger of physical assault. Nevertheless, parents often retrospectively realize that the child was giving messages of concern which the parents overlooked. In some instances, the child feigns physical illness just before the parents are to leave. Understandably, parents sometimes respond less than sympathetically, which only increases their sense of guilt when the true facts become known. In other instances, the child simply requests another babysitter but is vague and noncommittal when asked the reasons for his change in views. Professionals will immediately note the similarity between such behavior and that of young female children enmeshed in an incestuous relationship with an older male figure.

When the facts of the sexual assault become known, the parents of both the victim and the assailant are faced with a serious crisis. It is recommended that such parents contact rape crisis services and seek additional counseling if necessary. The parents of the victim frequently vacillate between rage at the assailant and guilt for having initiated the use of a male babysitter. Parents of assailants vacillate between the need to deny and an overwhelming sense of shame. Although the impact of such an experience on a young male child cannot be underestimated, it is quite likely that the long-term consequences are greatly influenced by the response of the parents to the situation, a response which can be modulated and handled more objectively with the help of professionals.

Male Rape in Prison

Rape of one inmate by another is an acknowledged fact of prison life. Fear of rape is one of the most commonly expressed concerns of young males convicted of criminal offenses and facing prison terms. This fear is particularly acute among young males who are small in stature, come from middle class backgrounds (thus often unsure of their ability to defend themselves), and/or have committed offenses that are despised by the average inmate, e.g., incest and child molestation.

The dynamics of prison rape have been studied by a number of investigators (Davis, 1968; Sagarin, 1976). It appears that the psychological motivation of rape within prison is not dissimilar to the desire for power and control that often motivates rapists who assault women outside of prison. Moreover, rape is an effective method for establishing social status within the prison inmate population. Scacco (1975) points out in a recent monograph on prison rape that rape of white inmates by black inmates is one method of dealing with pent-up racial tensions and hostilities.

An important aspect of rape within institutions that has not been sufficiently addressed by other sources is rape of inmates who are mentally disturbed or mentally disabled. Two points should be emphasized. First, since homosexuality is commonplace in penal institutions, and since homosexuality and mental illness are not always conceived as separate issues by correctional officers, sexual relations between "normal" inmates and mentally disabled inmates are not as likely to be viewed as resulting from coercion. Mentally disabled or disordered inmates are particularly vulnerable victims because their complaints may not be given credence. They may be more vulnerable also to carefully planned seduction that eventually leads to forced sexual relations. Furthermore, in the author's opinion, over the next ten years, social and legal pressures may inadvertently lead to increased criminalization of the mentally ill and disabled. If this occurs, more vulnerable inmates will be confined; therefore, protection of these inmates from forced sexual assault must be vigorously addressed by correctional officers and professional staff.

TABLE 1. EXAMPLES OF RAPE COUNTERMEASURES DESIGNED TO REDUCE THE FREQUENCY OR SEVERITY OF INJURIES

FACTORS	PHASES		
	Pre-rape	Rape	Post-rape
Offender Behavior	Early identification and treatment	Deterrent effect of punishment	Treatment and re-habilitation
Victim Behavior	Avoidance of male strangers	Self-defense	Help-seeking
Social Environment	Attitudes toward women	Bystander respon-siveness	Attitudes toward vic-tims
Physical Environ-ment	Security devices	Defensible space	Proximity of rape crisis centers

Source: Dietz PE: Social factors in rapist behavior, in Rada RT (ed): *Clinical Aspects of the Rapist.* New York, Grune and Stratton, 1978. Reproduced by permission of Park E. Dietz, MD.

PREVENTION STRATEGIES

Dietz (1978) ends his review of social factors in rapist behavior by stating, "The available evidence indicates that rape is committed by men from lower status segments of the population, at times of maximum social interaction, in whatever places men and women meet, against any women who are available." Likewise, Groth and Burgess (1980) found that male victims "are assaulted where they live, work, travel, and relax."

Such conclusions do not leave us feeling sanguine about prevention strategies. As individual professionals, we are likely to feel frustrated when attempting to bring about a reduction in violent assaults. A necessary first step in understanding how we may impact on rape is to conceptualize rape countermeasures in an organized and systematic manner. Dietz has presented one such attempt (1978). Table 1 lists examples of rape countermeasures designed to reduce the frequency or severity of injuries.

Several possible prevention strategies can be applied to offender behavior through early detection and treatment during the pre-rape phase. There is also a prevention strategy applicable to treatment and rehabilitation during the post-rape phase.

As was mentioned earlier, a significant number of rapists indicate that they had a pre-rape history of various sexual deviations, including peeping, voyeurism, exhibitionism, and fetishism. Some of these rapists were actually apprehended by authorities when engaging in such behavior. Others had been seen by professionals when they had become involved as juveniles in other nonsexual antisocial conduct. Rarely were these men asked about their violent sexual fantasies or concerns about their conflicted sexual life by police, correctional officers, or mental health professionals. Many were dismissed with a "boys will be boys" attitude. Although their shame or fear prevented them from volunteering their sexual concerns, many wish that they had been asked about their sexual lives because they were eager for an opportunity to discuss their conflicts. Professionals who have worked with adolescents or juvenile delinquents know that discussions of their sexual feelings must be conducted with utmost tact and concern. Nevertheless, a thorough social history should include a careful sexual history which may reveal developing sexual conflicts susceptible to early psychotherapeutic intervention.

Related to juvenile deviations is the issue of progression from less violent to more violent sex offenses. It is true that patients exhibiting certain types of sexual paraphilias, such as exhibitionism, peeping, or fetishism, tend to be characterologically passive and nonviolent. Some, however, do progress to more violent offenses such as rape. Furthermore, certain rapists continue to engage in these nonviolent paraphilias during the same periods when they are committing rapes. Psychotherapists should be alert to these possibilities when performing initial diagnostic evaluations on sexual paraphiliacs and should also carefully monitor the violent proclivities of these patients during active treatment.

The author and his colleagues have recently conducted a detailed evaluation of men sent for pre-trial evaluation on charges of murder or assault and battery. Twenty-five men charged with murder and 56 men charged with assault and battery were studied and data were obtained on their history of rape fantasies and rape activity. Ten (11 percent) of the 81 men admitted to a history of rape fantasies. One murderer had a previous conviction for statutory rape and two of those charged with assault and battery admitted they had committed rape for which they were not apprehended. These data suggest that men charged with or incarcerated for nonsexual aggressive crimes should be screened regarding their sexual history and sexually aggressive tendencies.

A number of studies have indicated a high association between rape, alcoholism, and drinking at the time of the commission of the rape (Rada, 1975; Rada et al., 1978). Several theories have been proposed to explain how heavy drinking might influence the commission of sexual offenses (Rada, 1975a; Barnard et al., 1979). A high association between drinking and the commission of a sexual offense does not, of course, prove a cause-and-effect relationship. Nevertheless, it does appear that in some instances alcohol is a definite facilitating factor in the commission of a sexual offense or assault. Thus, it is imperative that rehabilitation of sex offenders include treatment not only for their sexual conflicts but also of their alcohol abuse or addiction.

These prevention strategies relate specifically to the offender during the pre-rape and post-rape phase. Although these strategies may eventually prove useful, the most effective treatments currently available are those that focus on injury prevention and early care of victims. This type of approach is best rendered by the continued active support of victims through resource services such as Rape Crisis Centers. Until we have a better understanding of the multiple factors motivating rapists' behavior, we should concentrate our attention on reducing the severity of injury through efforts directed at potential and actual victims.

ACKNOWLEDGMENTS

The author acknowledges the helpful advice and suggestions of Lynn Rosner, MA, Rebecca Jackson, MD, and Meri Richards, BSN.

REFERENCES

Abel GG, Barlow DH, Blanchard EB, Guild D: The components of rapists' sexual arousal. *Arch Gen Psychiatry* 34: 895–903, 1977

Barbaree HE, Marshall WL, Lanthier RD: Deviant sexual arousal in rapists. *Behav Res Ther* 17:215–222, 1979

Barnard GW, Holzer C, Hernan V: A comparison of alcoholics and non-alcoholics charged with rape. *Bull Am Acad Psychiatry Law* 7:432–440, 1979

Burgess AW, Holmstrom LL: *Rape: Victims of Crisis.* Bowie, Robert J Brady, 1974

Buss AH, Fischer H, Simmons AJ: Aggression and hostility in psychiatric patients. *J Consult Psychol* 26:84–89, 1962

Davis AJ: Sexual assaults in the Philadelphia prison system and sheriff's van. *Trans-Action* 6:8–16, 1968

Dietz PE: Social factors in rapist behavior, in Rada RT (ed): *Clinical Aspects of the Rapist.* New York, Grune and Stratton, 1978

Gebhard PH, Gagnon JH, Pomeroy WB, Christenson CV: *Sex Offenders.* New York, Harper & Row, 1965

Glueck BC: Psychodynamic patterns in the homosexual sex offender. *Am J Psychiatry* 112:584–589, 1956

Groth AN, Birnbaum HJ: *Men Who Rape: The Psychology of The Offender*. New York, Plenum Press, 1979

Groth AN, Burgess AW: Sexual dysfunction during rape. *N Engl J Med* 297:764–766, 1977

Groth AN, Burgess AW: Male rape: Offenders and victims. *Am J Psychiatry* 137:806–810, 1980

Karpman B: A case of paedophilia (legally rape) cured by psychoanalysis. *Psychoanal Rev* 37:235–276, 1950

Karpman B: *The Sexual Offender and His Offenses*. New York, The Julian Press, 1959

Kaufman A, Divasto P, Jackson R, et al.: Male rape victims: Noninstitutional assault. *Am J Psychiatry* 137:221–223, 1980

Rada RT: Alcohol and rape. *Med Asp Hum Sex* 9:48–65, 1975a

Rada RT: Alcoholism and forcible rape. *Am J Psychiatry* 132:444–446, 1975b

Rada RT: Commonly asked questions about the rapist. Medical Aspects of Human Sexuality 11:47–56, 1977

Rada RT: Psychological factors in rapist behavior, in Rada RT (eds): *Clinical Aspects of the Rapist*. New York, Grune and Stratton, 1978a

Rada RT: Sociopathy and alcohol abuse, in Reid WH (ed) *The Psychopath: A Comprehensive Study of Sociopathic Disorders and Behaviors*. New York, Brunner/Mazel, 1978b

Rada RT, Kellner R, Laws DR, Winslow WW: Drinking, alcoholism, and the mentally disordered sex offender. *Bull Am Acad Psychiatry Law* 6:296–300, 1978

Rada RT, Laws DR, Kellner R, et al.: Plasma testosterone, dihydrotestosterone, and luteinizing hormone in violent and nonviolent sex offenders, submitted for publication

Rada RT, Laws DR, Kellner R: Plasma testosterone levels in the rapist. *Psychosom Med* 38:257–268, 1976

Sagarin E: Prison homosexuality and its effect on post-prison sexual behavior. *Psychiatry* 39:245–257, 1976

Scacco AM: *Rape In Prison*. Springfield, Ill: Charles C Thomas, 1975

Shultz GD: *How Many More Victims?* Philadelphia, Lippincott, 1965

Wille WS: Case study of a rapist: An analysis of the causation of criminal behavior. *J Soc Ther* 7:10–21, 1961

4

Homosexuality and the Medical Model

Charles W. Socarides

INTRODUCTION

The definition of "homosexual" and "homosexuality" can well be preceded by definitions of "sexual," "heterosexual," and "heterosexuality."

Sexual reproduction was antedated by asexual reproduction or fission, that is, one cell splitting into two identical cells. The word *sexual* is derived from biology and refers to a form of reproduction occurring between two cells which are different from each other. Their combined nuclear material resulted in a completely new individual cell and this became the basis of all evolutionary development. Sexual development began solely as reproductive activity. Use of the term has been enlarged to include sexual pleasure activity with or without reproduction.

Heterosexual object choice is determined by 2½ billion years of human evolution, a product of sexual differentiation. At first based solely on reproduction, it later widened to include sexual gratification: from one-celled nonsexual fission to the development of two-celled sexual reproduction, to organ differentiation, and finally to the development of two separate individuals reciprocally adapted to each other anatomically, endocrinologically, psychologically, and in many other ways.

Portions of this article have appeared before in "Homosexuality" by Charles W. Socarides in AMERICAN HANDBOOK OF PSYCHIATRY, second edition, Volume III edited by Silvano Arieti and Eugene B. Brody. © 1974 by Basic Books, Inc. By permission of Basic Books, Inc. Publishers, New York.

In man heterosexual object choice is not innate or instinctual, nor is homosexual object choice: both are learned behavior. The choice of sexual object is not predetermined by chromosomal tagging. However, most significantly, heterosexual object choice is outlined from birth by anatomy and then reinforced by cultural and environmental indoctrination. It is supported by universal human concepts of mating and the tradition of the family unit, together with the complementary aspects of and contrast between the two sexes.

Everything from birth to death is designed to perpetuate the male-female combination. This pattern is not only culturally ingrained but anatomically outlined and fostered by all the institutions of marriage, society, and the deep roots of the family unit. The term "anatomically outlined" does *not* mean that it is instinctual to choose a person of the opposite sex (heterosexuality). The human being is a biological emergent entity derived from evolution favoring survival.

In man, due to the tremendous development of the cerebral cortex, motivation—both conscious and unconscious—plays a crucial role in the selection of individuals and/or objects that will produce sexual arousal and orgastic release. When massive childhood fears have damaged and disrupted the standard male-female pattern, the roundabout method of achieving orgastic release is through instituting male-male or female-female pairs (homosexuality). Early unconscious fears are responsible not only for the later development of homosexuality but of all other modified sexual patterns of the obligatory type.

The term "standard" was originated by Rado to signify penetration of the male organ into the female at some point before orgasm and, of course, carries with it the potential for reproduction. Within the standard pattern, from which the foregoing characteristics are never absent, there are innumerable variations dependent upon individual preference. Homosexuality is a modified pattern because it does not conform to the essential characteristics of the standard pattern. Other modified sexual patterns, also referred to as perversions or deviations, include fetishism, voyeurism, exhibitionism, and pedophilia. Individuals suffering from these conditions have in common the inability to perform in the standard male-female design and, as one of their aims, attempt to achieve orgastic release in a substitutive way. A homosexual is an individual who engages repetitively or episodically in sexual relations with a partner of the same sex or experiences the recurrent desire to do so. If required to function sexually with a partner of the opposite sex he can do so, if at all, only with very little or no pleasure.

In April 1973, a 15 page memorandum issued by a group of militant homosexual organizations began with the following statement:

> . . . We submit that the presently held "illness model" of homosexuality is unwarranted, inasmuch as homosexuality per se has no known "pathogenesis," no specific "presenting symptoms," no recognizable "course of illness," and certainly no consistent outcome or "cure."

This statement reflects arguments presented by some psychiatrists, eg, Marmor (1973), Stoller (1973), Spitzer (1973), Green (1973) and Hoffman (1968).

Marmor equated homosexuality with either left-handedness or vegetarianism; Stoller regards it as a sexual "preference" of conscious decision; Spitzer finds it an "irregular" sexual orientation without etiological psychodynamics; to Green it is of hereditary origins of a nature as yet undiscovered; Hoffman believes it represents merely one end of the Kinsey rating scale of *normal* sexual behavior ranging from exclusive heterosexuality to exclusive homosexuality. All of them agree that:

1. There is no psychiatric disorder producing homosexuality and the only conflicts in the condition, if any, arise from society's attitude and the inability of the homosexual to accept his "lot" in life (conflict-free theory of origin).

2. Homosexuality of the exclusive type simply constitutes a normal variation of sexual behavior.*

Similar notions are to be found in the position taken in the Wolfenden Report (1957), items 25 through 30. For example: homosexuality does not satisfy the three criteria of a disease "(1) the presence of abnormal symptoms, which are caused by (2) a demonstrable pathological condition, in turn caused by (3) some factor called 'the cause,' each link in this causal chain being understood as something necessarily antecedent to the next . . . The tendency to regard homosexuality as an illness is likely to be a manifestation of confusing illness with 'moral failure' with its implications of 'irresponsibility' . . . Homosexuality cannot legitimately be regarded as a disease because in many cases it is the only symptom and is compatible

---

*These two positions were subsequently embodied in an official action of the APA voting to delete homosexuality from the DSM 2, as in their view, it is simply "a form of sexual behavior, like other forms of sexual behavior which are not by themselves psychiatric disorders."

with full mental health in other respects . . . Homosexuality is not a disorder because 'the alleged psychopathological causes' adduced for homosexuality have, however, also been found to occur in others besides the homosexual."

In refutation of the foregoing contentions, it is still the widely held scientific position of the large majority of psychiatrists in the United States and elsewhere that exclusive homosexuality is pathological and further, that the medical model is applicable insofar as it can be viewed in terms of an emotional disorder of any category. In the author's view, the rationale for such conviction is fully supported by the considerations which follow.

ETIOLOGY

There are three theories as to the basis of homosexual object choice. The first, originally suggested by Freud, was that of constitutional bisexuality. This assumes that in addition to an innate constitutional sexual predisposition to opposite sex partners, there exists a similar unconscious and innate predisposition to same sex partners. Freud (1905) felt that man's bisexuality in interaction with experiential factors in childhood was responsible for the expression of one choice or the other. He later placed less emphasis on the constitutional factor, stating that we should note "the connection between the sexual instinct and the sexual object" is not as intimate as one would surmise. Both are merely "soldered together." He warned that we must loosen the conceptual bonds which exist between instinct and object: "It seems probable that the sexual instinct is in the first instance independent of its object nor is its origin likely to be due to the object's attraction." He unequivocally stated that in cases of exclusiveness of homosexual object choice it is correct to regard homosexuality as pathological.

Those who stress a basic biological, instinctually determined drive toward heterosexuality commit the same error as advocates of the theory of constitutional bisexuality. Rado (1940) puts "constitutional bisexuality" in its proper place: In both lines of experimental study, the available evidence points to the same conclusion: the human male and female do not inherit an organized neuro-hormonal machinery of courtship and mating. Nor do they inherit any organized component mechanism that would—or could—direct them to such goals as mating or choice of mate. In the light of this evidence, the psychoanalytic theory of sexual instincts evolved in the first decades of this century has become an historical expedient that has outlived its scientific usefulness. Each of the sexes has an innate capacity for learning, and is equipped with a specific power plant and tools. But in sharp contrast to the lower vertebrates, and as a consequence of the encephalization of certain functions first organized at lower evolutionary levels of the central nervous system, they inherit no organized information.

A second theory, as enunciated by Bieber (1962) holds that where reproduction depends on heterosexual mating, there are built-in mechanisms to guarantee heterosexual arousal and behavior. In mammals, these built-in mechanisms are largely mediated through olfaction. Evidence is accumulating, according to this source, that olfaction is operant in human sexual development. Neurological and humoral mechanisms in concert with experiential factors, under normal childhood conditions, guarantee heterosexual object choice. Failure of these mechanisms makes one prone to substitutive sexual arousal patterns.

In 1968, the author introduced the concept that in all obligatory homosexuals there has been an inability to make the progression from the mother-child unity of earliest infancy to individuation (preoedipal theory of causation) (Mahlep and Furer, 1968). This failure in sexual identity, normally occurring by the age of three, is due to a pathological family constellation in which there is a domineering, psychologically crushing mother who will not allow the child to achieve autonomy from her and an absent, weak, or rejecting father who is unable to aid the son to overcome the block in maturation. As a result there exists in homosexuals a partial fixation with the concomitant tendency to regression to the earliest mother-child relationship (Socarides, 1968).

It is my belief, following Rado's model (1950), that all disordered behavior begins with an overproduction of fear, rage, guilt, and pain, the first clinical manifestations of which are found in early childhood. If sustained, these reactions produce an inhibition in performance, behavior, and productive potential of the organism. The latter responds by moves of misguided repair (symptom formation). Psychosexual disorders are no exception to the formula.

PSYCHOPATHOLOGY

Pathology, whether somatic or psychic, is defined as failure of function with concomitant pain and/ or suffering. It is this failure, its significance, and its manifold consequences which are so obvious in obligatory pre-oedipal homosexuality—a failure in functioning which, if carried to its extreme, would mean the death of the species.

A number of items serve as indicators of psychic pathology in the obligatory homosexual. They may not all appear in all cases and they may differ qualitatively and quantitatively from patient to patient. Some of those most commonly found are*:

1. A lifelong persistence of the original primary feminine identification with the mother and a consequent sense of deficiency concerning one's masculine identity. The end result is a pervasive feeling of femininity or a deficient sense of masculinity.

2. A persistence of archaic and primitive psychic mechanisms, e.g., the presence of incorporative and projective anxieties.

3. Intense and impulsive qualities to the homosexual act. The homosexual act itself may be likened to the effects of the opium alkaloids in their magical restorative powers: the optimum "fix," reinstating the body ego and sense of self against a threat of disruption and, in severe cases, imminent disintegration of the personality. The homosexual act, therefore, derives its urgency from the emergency need of survival for the ego of the homosexual.

4. The dramatic appearance of severe anxiety, tension, depression, paranoidal fears, and other symptomatology upon attempting interruption of homosexual activities, therefore underscoring a function of the homosexual symptom: that it is a compromise formation against deep anxieties. This outcome of such interruption is consistently seen in the course of treating homosexuals in depth.

CLINICAL SYMPTOMS AND COURSE

In addition to the items set forth under the preceding section of psychopathology, a partial listing of the symptomatology of obligatory homosexuality is outlined below†:

1. Symptoms arising out of the failure to make the intrapsychic separation from the mother:

  a. Excessive clinging to the mother in infancy and early childhood.

  b. Severe anxiety upon separation from her, noticeable from earliest

---

*For complete listing, see Socarides CW: Homosexuality, in Arieti S and Brody EB (eds): *American Handbook of Psychiatry*, ed 2. New York, Basic Books, 1974.

†For complete listing, see Socarides CW: Homosexuality, in Arieti S and Brody EB (eds): New York, Basic Books, 1974.

childhood ("screaming phenomenon") and continuing throughout life.

   c. Merging and fusion phenomena, fear of the engulfing mother, faulty body ego image because of the failure to separate and the lack of delineation of one's own body from that of the mother. There may be a consequent inability to appreciate body-space relationships.

   d. Intensification of primary feminine identification.

2. Symptoms arising from the predominance of archaic primitive psychic mechanisms:

   a. Incorporative anxieties (fears of swallowing parts of one's own body, fears of internalized harmful objects, etc).

   b. Projective anxieties (paranoidal anxieties, e.g., fears of poisoning, bodily attack, and persecution).

3. Symptoms arising from faulty gender identity:

   a. Continuation of the persistence of primary feminine identification with the mother (inner feelings of femininity).

   b. Corresponding feelings of a deficit in masculinity with anxiety appearing when faced with attempted performance in the appropriate gender role.

4. Symptoms arising from the wish for and fear of extreme closeness to the mother, the intense dependency on her for a feeling of well-being and survival, and the intense identification with her:

   a. Intense oral-sadistic relationship with the mother (intense sadism toward her is disguised by its opposite, a masochistic attitude toward her).

   b. Passive homosexual feelings toward the father, often repressed (taking the place of the mother in sexual intercourse both to protect and supplant her and to wreak vengeance on the father through appropriating his penis).

   c. Maintenance of a position of optimal distance from and / or closeness to the mother and other women.

   d. Fear of the sudden approach of the mother as if she will devour, engulf, and incorporate him. (This fear of the mother's engulfment and control, which in part reflects his wish and dread of her domination, is then generalized to a fear of all women and engulfment by them especially by the female genitalia and pubic hair.)

5. Symptoms present in adulthood:

   a. Constant yearning and search for masculinity. Engaging in homosexual acts incorporates the male partner and his penis, thus "strengthening" himself.

b. A concern in every homosexual encounter with first disarming the partner through one's seductiveness, appeal, power, prestige, effeminacy or "masculinity." This simulation of the male-female pattern (active vs passive, the one who penetrates vs the one who is penetrated) should not lead to the conclusion that the major motivation of either partner is to achieve femininity; both partners are intent upon acquiring masculinity from each other. To disarm in order to defeat is the motif and if one submits in "defeat," gratification is nevertheless obtained by the victim vicariously through identification with the victor. Despite any surface manifestations to the contrary, no matter the degree of apparent affection, *to disarm and defeat* invariably is the predominant conscious and/or unconscious characteristic of all encounters between homosexuals.

c. Severe anxiety, fears of engulfment, a sense of bodily disintegration, and other regressive symptomatology resulting from premature attempts at sexual relations with women. It must be remembered that the homosexual act "magically" produces a psychic equilibrium in order to temporarily withstand the multiple anxieties which beset the homosexual.

CLASSIFICATION

Nearly 70 years ago Freud (1905) proposed a classification based on both conscious and unconscious motivation:

1. Absolute inverts whose sexual objects are exclusively of their own sex and who are incapable of carrying out the sexual act with a person of the opposite sex or derive any enjoyment from it.

2. Amphigenic inverts whose sexual objects may equally well be of their own sex or of the opposite sex because this type of inversion lacks the characteristic of exclusiveness.

3. Contingent inverts, who take as their sexual objects those of their sex when circumstances preclude accessibility to partners of the opposite sex.

Current research has prompted this author to outline five major types of homosexuality as follow.*

*Acknowledgment is made here of this author's indebtedness to Rado (1949) for his original concepts of reparative, situational, and variational homosexuality.

1. Pre-oedipal Type
   a. This type is due to a *fixation* in the pre-oedipal phase of development (birth to three years of age).
   b. It is unconsciously motivated and arises from anxiety. Because nonengagement in homosexual practices results in intolerable anxiety and because the partner must be of the same sex it may be termed obligatory homosexuality. This sexual pattern is inflexible and stereotyped.
   c. Severe gender identity disturbance is present: In the male, a faulty and weak masculine identity; in the female, a faulty, distorted, and unacceptable feminine identity derived from the mother who is felt to be hateful and hated.
   d. Sexual identity disturbance is due to a persistence of the *primary feminine identification* as a result of the inability to traverse the separation-individuation phase (1½–3 years of age) and develop a separate and independent identity from the mother. In the female there persists an identification with the hated mother which she must reject. It is essential here to differentiate between primary and secondary feminine identification. Following the birth of the child the biological oneness with the mother is replaced by a primitive identification with her. The child must proceed from the security of identification and oneness with the mother to active competent separateness: in the boy toward active male [phallic] strivings, in the female, to active feminine strivings. If this task proves too difficult, pathological defenses, especially an increased aggressiveness, may result. These developments are of the greatest importance for the solution of conflicts appearing in the oedipal phase and in later life. In the boy's oedipal phase, under the pressure of the castration fear, an additional type of identification— secondary identification—with the mother in a form of passive feminine wishes for the father is likely to take place. However, beneath this feminine position in relation to the father one may often uncover the original passive relation with the mother, i.e., an active feminine pre-oedipal primary identification. In the oedipal phase of the girl, fear emanating from both parents—a conviction of rejection by the father because she is a female and by the mother because the latter is hateful and hated—leads to a secondary identification. This results in passive feminine wishes for the mother and in a masculine identification superimposed on the girl's deeper hated feminine identification in order to secure the "good" mother [the female homosexual partner later in life.]

e. The anxieties which beset persons of this type are of an insistent and intractable nature leading to an overriding, almost continual search for sexual partners.

f. There is persistence of primitive and archaic mental mechanisms leading to an abundance of incorporation and projection anxieties.

g. The anxiety which develops is due to fears of engulfment, ego dissolution, and loss of self and ego boundaries. The homosexual act is needed to ensure ego survival and transiently stabilize the sense of self. Consequently, the act must be repeated frequently out of inner necessity to ward off paranoidal and incorporative fears. (The rare exceptions in this type who cannot consciously accept the homosexual act struggle mightily against it and, therefore, the symptom remains latent as explained in the fifth type—latent).

h. The homosexual symptom is *ego-syntonic* as the nuclear conflicts, e.g., fears of engulfment, loss of ego boundaries, loss of self, have undergone a transformation and disguise through the mechanism of the repressive compromise, allowing the more acceptable part of infantile sexuality to remain in consciousness.

i. There is a predominance of pre-genital characteristics of the ego; remembering is often replaced by acting out.

j. The aim of the homosexual act is ego survival and a reconstitution of a sense of sexual identity in accordance with anatomy. The male achieves "masculinity" through identification with the male sexual partner; the act reassures against and lessens castration fear. The female achieves "resonance" identification with the woman partner; the act reassures against and lessens castration fears. She also creates the "good" mother-child relationship.

2. Oedipal Type

a. This type is due to a failure to resolve the oedipus complex and from castration fears leading to the adoption of a negative oedipal position and a *regression* in part to anal and oral conflicts (a partial pre-oedipal regression). The male assumes the role of the female with the father (other men); the female assumes the role of the male to the mother (other women).

b. Homosexual wishes in this type are unconsciously motivated and dreaded; engagement in homosexual practices is not obligatory. The sexual pattern is flexible in that heterosexuality can be carried out and is usually the conscious choice.

c. Gender identity disturbances of masculine sexual identity in the male (or deficient feminine sexual identity in the female) are due to a *secondary identification* with a person (parent) of the opposite sex in this type. (This is simply a reversal of normal sexual identification in the direction of the same-sex parent.)

d. The anxiety which develops in the male is due to fears of penetration by the more powerful male (father); the female fears rejection by the more powerful female (mother). Common to both are shame and guilt arising from superego and ego conflicts, conscious and unconscious, attendant to engaging in homosexual acts in dreams and fantasies and, occasionally, in actuality under special circumstances of stress. Homosexual acts in this type are attempts to ensure dependency and attain power through the seduction of the more powerful partner.

e. Primitive and archaic psychic mechanisms may appear due to *regression*. These are intermittent and do not lend a stamp of pregenitality to the character traits of the individual as in the pre-oedipal type.

f. The homosexual symptom is *ego-alien*. Although unconsciously determined, it is not the outcome of the repressive compromise as described in Type One above. The symptom may remain at the level of unconscious thoughts, dreams, and fantasies as it is not a disguised acceptable representation of a deeper conflict. When it threatens to break into awareness, anxiety develops. However, under certain conditions, e.g., defiant rage overriding the restraining mechanism of conscience or periods of intense depression secondary to loss with resultant needs for love, admiration, and strength from a person of the same sex, homosexual acts may take place. Such acts, however, do not achieve the magical symbolic restitution of the pre-oedipal type. They may instead exacerbate the situation through loss of pride and self-esteem.

g. The aim of the homosexual act is to experience dependency on and security from "powerful" figures of the same sex. The sexual pattern of the negative oedipal type is not as inflexible or stereotyped as in the pre-oedipal type. There are exacerbations and remissions in the sense of masculine identity (in the female in the sense of pride and achievement in feminine identity) secondary to successful performance in other (nonsexual) areas of life. Such feelings of success diminish any fantasied or actual need for sexual relations with persons of the same sex.

3. Situational Type
   a. Environmental inaccessibility to partners of the opposite sex is present.
   b. The behavior is consciously motivated.

    c. Homosexual acts are not fear-induced but arise out of conscious deliberation and choice.

    d. The person is able to function with a partner of the opposite sex.

    e. The sexual pattern is flexible and these individuals do return to opposite sex partners when they are available.

4. Variational Type

    a. The motivations underlying this form of homosexual behavior are as varied as the motivations which drive men and women to pursue power, gain protection, assure dependency, seek security, wreak vengeance, or experience specialized sensations. In some cultures such surplus activity is a part of the established social order; in others, it is entirely a product of individual enterprise contrary to the general social order. The homosexuality practiced in ancient Greece was in all probability variational in type. There were strict laws against it (except for its practice during a brief period in late adolescence). Penalties included disenfranchisement of those engaged in catamite activities (anal intercourse). Sentiments expressing admiration and affection for youth (so-called homosexual sentiments) short of homosexual relations in ancient Greece were allowed. In ancient Sparta homosexuality could be punished by death.

    b. The behavior is consciously motivated.

    c. Homosexual acts are not fear-induced but arise out of conscious deliberation and choice.

    d. The person is able to function with a partner of the opposite sex.

    e. The sexual pattern is flexible and these individuals do return to opposite sex partners when they so prefer.

5. Latent Type

    a. This type has the underlying psychic structure of either the pre-oedipal or oedipal type (Types One and Two) without homosexual practices.

    b. There is much confusion in the use of the term "latent homosexuality" due to the erroneous and outmoded concept of constitutional bisexuality. This implies that side-by-side with an innate desire for partners of the opposite sex, there exists an inborn or innate desire for same-sex partners. Correctly, latent homosexuality means the presence in an individual of the underlying psychic structure of either the pre-oedipal or oedipal type without overt orgastic activity with a person of the same sex.

    c. The shift from latent to overt and the reverse is dependent on several factors: (1) The strength of the fixation at the pre-oedipal level (quantitative factor), severity of anxiety, and the intensity of regression from the later oedipal conflict; (2) The acceptability of the homosexuality to the ego (self), the superego (conscience mechanism), and the ego ideal; and (3) The strength of the instinctual drives, i.e., libido and aggression. These individuals may never or rarely engage in overt homosexual activities.

d. The latent homosexual may or may not have any conscious knowledge of his preference for individuals of the same sex for orgastic fulfillment. On the other hand, there may be a high degree of elaboration of unconscious homosexual fantasies and homosexual dream material with or without conscious denial of its significance. They may live an entire lifetime without realizing their homosexual propensities, managing to function marginally on a heterosexual level, sometimes getting married and having children.

e. Another pattern is that of the individual who, fully aware of his homosexual preference, abstains from all homosexual acts. Others, as a result of severe intolerable stress, infrequently and transiently engage in overt homosexual acts, living the major portion of their lives, however, as latent homosexuals. In the latent phase they may maintain a limited heterosexual functioning, albeit unrewarding, meager, and usually based on homosexual fantasies. Or they may utilize homosexual fantasy for masturbatory practices or may abstain from sexual activity altogether. These individuals are, of course, truly homosexual at all times; the shift between latent and overt and the reverse constitutes an alternating form of latent homosexuality.

f. All forms of latent homosexuality are potentially overt. Social imbalance—where severe inequities exist between one's survival needs due to the failure of society to ensure their adequate satisfaction—has a precipitating effect in some borderline and/or latent cases of both pre-oedipal and oedipal homosexuality. Such imbalance also brings a flight from the female on the part of the male, a flight from all aspects of masculine endeavor, and a retreat to a less demanding role. This is a possible explanation of the apparent rise in the incidence of male homosexuality during periods of social turbulence when many traditional roles, privileges, and responsibilities are overturned. The same factors may cause an increase in female homosexuality.

DISCUSSION

Pre-oedipal and oedipal homosexuality are reparative in nature and "ushered in by the inhibition of standard performance through early [childhood] fears" (Rado, 1949). Pre-oedipal homosexuality may be compared to the narcotic addict's need for a "fix." The purpose of the homosexual act is to maintain the equilibrium of a highly disturbed individual.

Regarding the situational type, Bieber reported that, with rare exceptions, men who had not been homosexual prior to military service were found not to have engaged in homosexual activity throughout their tour of duty despite the absence of female partners (personal communication, 1973). This finding suggests a possible revision of the concept of situational homosexuality in instances where the coercive factor is absent. Much of the so-called situational factor in prisons is an outcome of the struggle for dominance and is, in fact, rape. The infrequency of validated situations in which heterosexuals engage in homosexual relations reaffirms the strength of the male-female design once established in the human psyche; parenthetically it explains the popularity of the "pin-up" during World War II. Undoubtedly, sexual outlet was achieved under those trying conditions of sexual deprivation via masturbation abetted by photographs of artistically posed semi-nude women.

Variational homosexuality may occur in individuals who seek to gratify the desire for an alternation of sexual excitation, often for reasons of impotence or near-impotence in the male partner of the heterosexual pair. Much of the heterosexual group sex activity currently reported includes homosexual behavior between male and female participants and is of this type. In some instances, individuals with unconsciously derived homosexual conflicts take part in such group activities in order to act out their homosexual wishes and simultaneously to deny their homosexual problem.

Variational homosexuality may also be seen in the neurotic, psychotic, and sociopath. It frequently occurs in those suffering from alcoholism as well as in depressive states.

THERAPY

It is now widely agreed that to achieve therapeutic success it is necessary to interpret to the patient his fear of castration, his fear of oral dependence, his distrust of the opposite sex, and his fear of his own destructiveness and sadism. However, in this writer's experience, the interpretation that most effectively achieves a relaxation of his resistance is that the homosexual act is an attempt to acquire masculinity through identification with the partner and his penis (Socarides, 1969, Freud, 1954). After this interpretation is worked through the patient may be able to function heterosexually, often going through a strong narcissistic-phallic phase, with women serving only the "grandeur" of his penis.

Detailed reports of successful resolution of cases of overt homosexuality have been published by Flournoy (1953), Lagache (1953), Poe (1952), Socarides (1969), Vinchon and Nacht (1931), and Wulff (1941). In addition, important insights are offered by Bergler (1956), Bychowski (1945, 1954, 1956), Anna Freud (1951); Sigmund Freud (1922), Glover (1933), Lorand (1956), Nunberg (1938), Ovesey (1969), Rosenfeld (1965), and Sachs (1923).

Data on positive therapeutic outcome have been collected in surveys by the American Psychoanalytic Association (1956), the Portman Clinic in London (1960), both primarily in statistical format, and by the Bieber study conducted by the Society of Medical Psychoanalysts (1962).

The central issues which must be uncovered and worked through by the patient are:

1. While the analysis of oedipal fears of incest and aggression is of paramount importance in the course of treatment, it is vital to the understanding and successful resolution of homosexuality that the nuclear pre-oedipal anxieties be revealed. These consist of primitive fears of incorporation, threatened loss of personal identity, engulfment by the mother, and personal dissolution which would accompany any attempt to separate from her.

2. The homosexual makes an identification with his partner in the sexual act. Homosexual contact promotes a transient, pseudo-strengthening of his own masculinity and identity which must constantly be repeated or a psychic decompensation occurs. The homosexual seeks masculinity not feminity, and knowledge of this unconscious motivation becomes a potent source of strength, reassurance, and determination for change in the direction of homosexual functioning.

3. The conditions under which the imperative need for homosexual relief occurs include mounting anxiety, depression, and paranoid-type fears.

4. The ubiquitous presence of a distorted body ego is manifest.

5. The penis of the partner is revealed to be a substitute for the feed-

ing breast of the sought after "good" mother (breast = penis equation). The homosexual thereby escapes the frustrating cruel mother and makes up for the oral deprivation suffered at her hands.

6. There is a characteristic demeaning and degrading of the father, often quite openly. The patient identifies with the aggressor (mother). This hatred of the father produces guilt and in therapy is an impediment to his feeling of being entitled to be a man.

7. At unconscious levels there exists an intense yearning for the father's love and protection. This deprivation is a further frustration of the need for masculine identification. The homosexual act dramatizes the yearning as well as the frustration-derived aggression toward all men as a consequence.

8. Heterosexual interest and strivings are continually subject to suppression and repression in the course of therapy. This is due to unconscious guilt feelings toward the mother because of intense incestuous and aggressive impulses.

9. The careful maintenance of the positive therapeutic alliance is a considerable source of strength to the patient in his attempts to control and finally triumph over his fears of murderous retaliation on the part of the mother as he gradually moves toward his long sought after masculine identity.

Successful results utilizing group therapy have been reported by Gershman (1967), Hadden (1958, 1966), and T. Bieber (1971). Because the exploration of conscious and unconscious fantasies, feelings, and actions is limited in group therapy, it is wise to combine it with individual therapy.

CONCLUSION

My findings reveal, as do those of the researchers noted above, that homosexuality has an etiology, symptomatology, and course of development, and in most cases responds well to appropriate therapeutic techniques. Thus, as a psychiatric disorder, it follows that if all punitive and persecutory laws were banished immediately—as indeed they should be—the suffering which arises from this condition would not stop. Those who advocate declaring homosexuality "normal" betray the fundamental criterion of modern medicine which is devoted to correct diagnosis.

There is every reason to believe that since Freud first opened the door to treatment of the homosexual, offering the first opportunity for understanding and proper therapy of this complex condition, hope was offered to many who had often surrendered to despair. So it is today: the very real hope is that a favorable prognosis is quite possible in most cases when homosexuals choose to seek help.

REFERENCES

American Psychoanalytic Association: *Report of the Central Fact Gathering Committee.* New York, 1956, unpublished

Beagler E: *Homosexuality: Disease or Way of Life?* New York, Hill and Wang, 1956

Bieber I et al.: *Homosexuality: A Psychoanalytic Study of Male Homosexuals.* New York, Basic Books, 1962

Bieber T B: Group therapy with homosexuals, in Kaplan H I, Sadock B S (eds): *Comprehensive Group Therapy.* Baltimore, Williams and Wilkins, 1971

Bychowski G: The ego of homosexuals. *Int J Psychoanal* 26:114–127, 1945

Bychowski G: The structure of homosexual acting out. *Psychoanal Q* 23:48–61, 1954

Bychowski G: The Ego and the Introjects. *Psychoanal Q* 25:11–36, 1956

Flournoy H: An Analytic Session in a Case of Male Homosexuality. In Loewenstein R M (ed): *Drives, Affects, Behavior.* New York, International Universities Press, 1953

Freud A: Homosexuality. *Bull Am Psychoanal Assoc* 7:117–118, 1951

Freud A: Problems of technique in adult analysis. *Bull Philadelphia Assoc Psychoanal* 4:44–70, 1954

Freud S: *Three essays on the theory of sexuality. Standard Edition* 7:125–245, 1905

Freud S: *Some neurotic mechanisms in jealousy, paranoia and homosexuality. Standard Edition* 18:221–235, 1922

Gershman H: The evolution of gender identity. *Am J Psychoanal* 28:80–91, 1967

Glover E: The relation of perversion formation to the development of reality sense. *Int J Psychoanal* 14:486–504, 1933

Glover E: *The Roots of Crime: Selected Papers on Psychoanalysis,* vol 2. London, Imago Publishing, 1960

Green R: Should heterosexuality be in the APA nomenclature? Read before the Annual Meeting of the American Psychiatric Association, Hawaii, May 1973

Hadden S B: Treatment of homosexuality by individual and group psychotherapy. *Am J Psychiatry* 114:810–821, 1958

Hadden S B: Treatment of male homosexuals in groups. *Int J Group Psychother* 16:13–21, 1966

Hoffman M: *The Gay World.* New York, Basic Books, 1968

Lagache D: De l'homosexualité à la jalousie. *Rev Fr Psychoanal* 13:351–366, 1953

Lorand S: The Therapy of Perversions, in Lorand S, Balint M (eds): *Perversions: Psychodvnamics and Therapy.* New York, Random House, 1956

Mahle P M S, Furer M: *On Human Symbiosis and the Vicissitudes of Individuation.* New York, International Universities Press, 1968

Marmor J: Homosexuality and cultural value systems. Read before the Annual Meeting of the American Psychiatric Association, Hawaii, May 1973

Nunberg H: Homosexuality, magic, and aggression. *Int J Psychoanal* 19:1–16, 1938

Ovesey L: *Homosexuality and Pseudohomosexuality.* New York, Science House, 1969

Poe J S: The successful treatment of a 40-year-old passive homosexual based on an adaptational view of sexual behavior. *Psychoanal Rev* 39:23–33, 1952

Rado S: A critical examination of the concept of bisexuality. *Psychosom Med* 2:459–467, 1940

Rado S: An adaptational view of sexual behavior, in Hoch P H, Zubin J (eds): *Psychosexual Development in Health and Disease.* New York, Grune and Stratton, 1949

Rado S: Emergency behavior, with an introduction to the dynamics of conscience, in Hoch P H, Zubin J (eds): *Anxiety* New York, Grune and Stratton, 1950

Rosenfeld H A: *Psychotic States.* New York, International Universities Press, 1965

Sachs H: On the genesis of sexual perversion. *Int Z Psychoanal* 9:172–182, 1923. Bernays H F (trans): New York Psychoanalytic Institute Library, 1964

Socarides C W: A provisional theory of etiology in male homosexuality: A case of pre-oedipal origin. *Int J Psychoanaly* 49:27–37, 1968

Socarides C W: Psychoanalytic therapy of a male homosexual. *Psychoanal Q* 38:173–190, 1969

Spitzer R L: Should homosexuality be in the APA nomenclature? Read before the Annual Meeting of the American Psychiatric Association, Hawaii, May 1973

Stoller R J: Criteria for psychiatric diagnoses. Read before the Annual Meeting of the American Psychiatric Association, Hawaii, May 1973

Vinchon J, Nacht S: Considerations sur la cure psychanalytique d'ene nérvose homosexuelle. *Rev Fr Psychoanal* 4:677–709, 1931

Wolfenden J: *Report of the Committee on Homosexual Offences and Prostitution.* London, Her Majesty's Stationery Offices, 1957

Wulff M: Ueber einen fall von männlicher homosexualität. *Int Z Psychoanal* 26:105–121, 1941

5

Diagnostic Evaluation of Male Impotence: Problems and Promises

Ismet Karacan, Cengiz Aslan, and Robert L. Williams

Medical interest in the diagnostic evaluation of psychosexual disorders has accelerated in the past decade to keep pace with growing public demands for effective treatments of various sexual problems. As sexual awareness increased and sociocultural taboos against the scientific study of sexual disorders decreased, new, readily available techniques for managing such disorders were widely publicized. Kinsey became a household word and the work of Masters and Johnson the popular topic at cocktail parties. In this climate of growing optimism, impotent men, in particular, were lured "out of the closet" by promises of relief ranging from behavioral therapy to implantation of a penile prosthesis. Male impotence captured the medical research spotlight not only because its disruption of normal sexual functioning is global, but also because so little was known about its etiology.

The Diagnostic and Statistical Manual of Mental Disorders (DSM III) (American Psychiatric Association, 1980) classifies impotence as "recurrent and persistent inhibition of sexual excitement during sexual activity, manifested (in males) by partial or complete failure to attain or maintain erection until completion of the sexual act." Impotence, like other psychosexual dysfunctions, may be lifelong (primary) or acquired after a period of normal functioning (secondary), generalized or situational (limited to certain situations or partners), total or partial. The clinician must determine that the patient engages in sexual activity that is adequate in focus, intensity, and duration for erection to occur. Impotence is not classified as inhibited sexual excitement if the disturbance is caused exclusively by organic factors, such as a disease process or medication (Axis III), or by another major mental disorder (Axis I).*

These diagnostic criteria emphasize the importance of accurate differential diagnosis. Until recently, 90 percent of impotence was considered to be psychogenic rather than organogenic in etiology (Cooper, 1970; Hastings, 1963; Masters and Johnson, 1970; Strauss, 1950; Wershub, 1959). We believe that this assumption was based on an outdated diagnostic procedure that was incapable of detecting all possible relevant physical pathology. Too often, psychogenic impotence was diagnosed by default; a physician unable to discover a disease process typically associated with impotence, such as diabetes mellitus, automatically assumed a psychological etiology without positive evidence of mental disturbance.

The human and economic costs of inaccurate diagnosis have been high. The patient reporting a disillusioning 20-year history of trying one inappropriate and expensive treatment after another with no improvement is not an unusual finding at our diagnostic center.

Over the past 18 years, we have developed a procedure for evaluating impotence which emphasizes a crucial diagnostic tool—the monitoring of nocturnal penile tumescence (NPT)—in determining whether penile erection is physically possible. The DSM III manual states that "the measurement of nocturnal penile tumescence associated with REM sleep is a useful diagnostic technique for evaluating the degree to which a physical disorder is etiologically related to [inhibited sexual excitement]." We further contend that NPT monitoring should be a mandatory step in the diagnostic evaluation of every man who seeks medical or psychiatric treatment for impotence.

PREVALENCE OF IMPOTENCE

The current prevalence of impotence is uncertain, largely due to inconsistencies in methodology and in differentiating types of sexual complaints, inaccurate differential diagnoses, and failure to allow for age differences

---

*DSM III is a multiaxial evaluation in which every patient is assessed on three official diagnostic axes and, when indicated, on two supplementary axes designed for planning treatment and predicting outcome. Axis I refers to clinical syndromes, Axis II to personality and specific developmental disorders, and Axis III to physical disorders and conditions.

(Levins, 1976). That impotence increases with age, particularly after age 40, is well substantiated (Finkel et al., 1959; Verwoerdt et al., 1968; Pearlman and Kobashi, 1972; Pfeiffer et al., 1972); Kinsey et al (1948) found that 75 percent of men are impotent at age 80, whereas only 2 percent become impotent by age 40. More patients seek treatment for erectile difficulties than for other sexual problems such as loss of sexual desire or ejaculatory difficulty (Cooper, 1972; Masters and Johnson, 1970; Johnson, 1965; Raboch, 1970; Teoh and Lee, 1974). At high risk of developing erectile failure are patients with multiple sclerosis, paraplegia, vascular diseases, certain psychoses, diabetes mellitus, and end-stage renal disease. About 50 percent of patients who have had adult-onset diabetes mellitus for six years or longer (Karacan et al, 1978c), and between 33–100 percent of those with end-stage renal disease undergoing dialysis (Karacan et al., 1978a), suffer from impotence.

CAUSES OF IMPOTENCE

Impotence may have a primarily organogenic, psychogenic, or mixed etiology. Considering the growing evidence that "almost any physical dysfunction that reduces body economy below acceptable levels of metabolic efficiency can result in the onset of erective impotence" (Masters and Johnson, 1970), differential diagnosis becomes an awesome task. At least 100 organic conditions of the cardiovascular, endocrine, genitourinary, hematologic, neural, and respiratory systems, as well as certain drugs (eg, alcohol, antihypertensives, antipsychotics, tricyclic antidepressants) and various psychological conditions, may produce impotence. Organic conditions that typically contribute to impotence are diabetes mellitus, arteriosclerosis, prostatectomy or abdominal perineal resection, trauma to the penis or spinal cord, Peyronie's disease, priapism, and CNS lesions. For a more comprehensive list of such conditions by system, see Karacan et al. (1978c).

Nearly every psychological condition—psychosis, depression, anxiety, personality characteristics—has been associated with impotence, yet only functional psychoses and inverted sex drive have been clinically assigned definite etiological significance (Cooper, 1969). In DSM III, the American Psychiatric Association (APA) links inhibited sexual excitement to compulsive traits as well as to any negative attitude toward sexuality. The APA also implicates depression, anxiety, guilt, shame, frustration, and somatic symptoms. Although psychogenic factors should be recognized, most of the evidence for their association with impotence derives from case studies and theoretical discussions rather than from systematic research. Further complicating the identification of causal factors is the physician's tendency to assume an either/or etiology when, actually, psychological and organic causes may coexist in the same patient. For example, the impotence of a patient exhibiting signs of anxiety and depression may have originally resulted from an unidentified organic deficit. Indeed, most impotent men, especially when the dysfunction has been long-standing, will show some reactionary emotional disturbance. Yet too often, the impotence is attributed exclusively to these secondary psychological factors.

FLAWS IN THE STANDARD DIAGNOSTIC PROCEDURE

The standard recommended procedure for differential diagnosis of impotence has not improved in over 30 years (Keshin and Pinek, 1949; Compere, 1978). The physician reviews the patient's medical history and performs a routine physical examination and standard laboratory tests to identify relevant physical pathology, and then examines the developmental history to identify indicators of psychological involvement such as: (1) rapid onset of impotence, (2) selective or transient occurrence of impotence, or (3) persistence of occasional masturbatory, morning, or other spontaneous erections (Simpson, 1950). Symptoms and signs of physical pathology denote organogenic impotence, positive findings in the developmental history psychogenic impotence, and the presence of both types a mixed etiology. In practice, however, the absence of clear signs or symptoms typically results in the default diagnosis of psychogenic impotence (Karacan and Salis, 1980).

Several deficits in this procedure make its validity questionable. Examination of the physical systems is inadequate because differential diagnosis depends on accurate detection of all physical pathology, but:

1. Routine examinations are not sufficient to explore all known relevant pathology.

2. The physiological mechanisms of normal human erection and impotence, largely extrapolated from studies of animals or diseased, injured or deceased humans are unknown.

3. Most cause-effect relationships between potential contributors and impotence are assumed rather than systematically proven, limiting definitive statements about etiology even for pathology widely accepted as relevant, such as diabetes or multiple sclerosis.

4. Examination of the patient's erect penis to verify his complaint of

impotence and to assess actual erectile capability is not included, yet certain relevant disease processes or structural abnormalities are not easily detected in the flaccid penis.

Similarly, the psychological evaluation has serious shortcomings. Accurate diagnosis depends upon the validity of an exclusive relationship between the psychological indicators and psychogenic impotence. However:

1. No systematic research demonstrates this validity; the psychological symptoms may also characterize certain types of organogenic impotence.

2. The psychological evaluation is even more superficial than the physical evaluaton, eg, objective psychological tests are rarely administered.

3. The psychological mechanisms of impotence are unknown, limiting examination and conclusions about the etiology.

4. Determining whether a positive psychological finding is a cause or an effect of the impotence is difficult.

5. Psychogenic impotence is the usual default diagnosis in the absence of positive findings.

Thus, the chief impediments to accurate differential diagnosis using the standard procedure are its reliance on insensitive methods of locating deficits presumed to be related to the patient's complaint and the failure to directly observe the patient's erection. Consequently, the patient's actual complaint—inadequate erection—is never directly examined, inaccurate diagnoses are common, and false-negative physical findings and false-positive psychological findings inevitably occur (Karacan and Salis, 1980). Moreover, the defects in the evaluation procedure invalidate the widely held belief that most impotence is psychogenic.

EVOLUTION OF AN OBJECTIVE DIAGNOSTIC TOOL: NPT

The limitations in the standard diagnostic procedure impelled us to explore a reliable indicator of erectile capacity. Because penile erection has been known since the 1940's to occur during sleep (Halverson, 1940; Ohlmeyer and Brilmayer, 1947; Ohlneyer et al., 1944), and in the following two decades had been associated with REM sleep (Jovanovic, 1967; Oswald, 1962; Shapiro, 1964), the phase characterized by autonomic activation and dreaming, monitoring of nocturnal penile tumescence (NPT) appeared to be a promising diagnostic tool for impotence. Further research confirmed that at least 80 percent of REM periods in young adult men are temporally associated with NPT (Fisher et al., 1965; Karacan, 1965; Karacan et al., 1966) and that NPT is a common phenomenon in infants, and middle-aged and elderly men (Jovanovic 1972; Kahn and Fisher, 1969a, 1969b; Karacan, 1966). If we could prove that NPT was a univeral phenomenon in normal men, the presence of nocturnal erections could serve as a "biological marker" for erectile capacity.

We subsequently designed a mercury-filled strain gauge (Karacan, 1969) to more accurately monitor penile circumference changes as a measure of NPT. Using this gauge, systematic studies of 125 healthy males aged 3–79 years revealed not only that NPT does indeed occur in all healthy males, but that it undergoes predictable quantitative and qualitative changes with age (Karacan et al., 1972b, 1972c; Hursch et al. 1972; Karacan et al., 1972a, 1975, 1976). The frequency and amount of NPT declined steadily from age 20, whereas the amount of REM-related NPT slightly, but consistently, increased with age. In the six adult age groups (20-79), an NPT episode began about every 72–100 minutes. The number of REM-related NPT episodes per night ranged from 3.9 at 20–29 years to 2.6 at 70–79 years.

None of the healthy potent men recorded since these ontogenetic studies have had significantly impaired or absent NPT. On the other hand, in clinical applications of NPT monitoring in men with medical conditions likely to impair erectile function, high percentages of men with diabetes (Karacan, 1970, 1980; Karacan et al., 1977b, 1978d, 1978e), alcoholism (Karacan et al., 1980a), end-stage renal disease (Karacan et al., 1978a), spinal cord injury (Karacan et al., 1977a; 1978b), and Shy-Drager syndrome (Moore et al., 1979) showed significant deficits in NPT. Such findings led to and support our basic assumption that NPT is a reliable index of physiological erectile capacity during the waking state, and to our working assumptions, for differential diagnosis, that impotence is psychogenic if the patient has normal NPT for his age and organogenic if NPT is abnormal for his age. Furthermore, follow-up evaluations of impotent patients to identify the specific pathology, now a routine part of the diagnostic evaluation of impotence, have supported our assumptions so far.

The following conclusions from our clinical experience validate NPT monitoring as a clinical diagnostic tool.

1. Most impotent men in whom the probability of organogenic impotence is high had impaired NPT.

2. Most impotent men in whom the probability of organogenic impotence is low had normal NPT.

3. Impotent men with impaired NPT benefited from corrections of contributory physiological deficits. For example, vascular surgery im-

proved the erectile functioning of men with impaired genital circulation (Karacan et al., 1978c; 1978e).

4. Behavioral or psychiatric treatment of impotence did not improve the erectile functioning of men with deficits in NPT. Men with diagnostic organogenic impotence who had contraindications to medical or surgical treatment were referred for behavioral or psychiatric treatment as the only available alternative. As expected, the treatment did not improve their potency or nocturnal erection (Karacan and Salis, 1980).

5. Impotent men with normal NPT did not respond well to medical treatment, but behavioral or psychiatric treatment improved erectile functioning. Patients with potentially contributory psychological disturbances who conscientiously completed the therapy program eventually experienced adequate potency (Karacan and Salis, 1980).

6. General or acute psychological factors did not significantly inhibit NPT. Although negative affect in REM dreams may produce transient NPT fluctuations (Karacan, 1965; Karacan et al., 1966; Fisher, 1966), NPT was not persistently altered by the psychological distress of severely neurotic men (Karacan and Salis, 1980).

7. Neither REM sleep irregularities nor frequency and proximity of sexual activity affected NPT. Several studies (Karacan and Salis, 1980; Karacan 1965; Fisher, 1966) showed that NPT continues to cycle in the normal manner when REM is suppressed. Furthermore, neither prolonged deprivation of orgasm followed by sexual satiation, nor sexual arousal without orgasm immediately before sleep, had significant effect on NPT (Karacan et al., 1970; 1979).

RECOMMENDED PROCEDURE FOR DIFFERENTIAL DIAGNOSIS OF IMPOTENCE

Over the past 18 years, we have evolved an objective procedure for the differential diagnosis of impotence. Due to its emphasis on NPT monitoring as a direct test for organic involvement, supplemented by measurements of neuromuscular and vascular function during waking and sleeping, our three-day evaluation procedure at the sleep disorders center adjusts for the deficiencies in the standard procedure. The procedure is designed to positively identify physical and psychological pathology; the former by examining physical, morphological, urological, neural and neuromuscular, and vascular and endocrine systems, and by checking on drug use, the latter through psychiatric interviews and psychological tests.

A one to two-hour intake interview designed to obtain a complete medical history and description of the presenting complaint is the first step in the diagnostic procedure. The interview focuses on the patient's developmental sexual and marital histories and current sexual functioning. The interviewer pays particular attention to the temporal development and exact nature of erectile dysfunction, the situations in which failure occurs, dynamic interaction with the partner, how the current level of sexual functioning compared to previous, typical levels, a history of medical conditions suspected of contributing to impotence, hospitalizations or treatment for psychiatric illness, present and past drug prescriptions, and possible alcohol or drug abuse. In addition, the family and social histories provide clues to diseases or situations possibly related to the presenting complaint. The temporal relationship between any conditions revealed in the interview and the onset or intensification of impotence is carefully noted. The intake interview is useful in exploring both the physical and psychological etiology of impotence.

EVALUATION OF PHYSICAL ETIOLOGY

A general physical examination of all major systems and standard laboratory tests follows the interview. The initial examination concentrates on morphological characteristics; the external genitalia are carefully examined for structural defects.

The neurological examination identifies impaired reflexes and motor or sensory deficits in the lower trunk and extremities. Failure of either the EKG-measured heart rate to correspondingly decelerate during one minute of deep, slow breathing or the pupils to contract in response to a sudden, bright light indicates disturbance in the autonomic nervous system. Penile sensory deficit and pelvic or penile pain are neurosensory problems that may compromise satisfactory intercourse yet often yield normal NPT results. Electrically induced, coronal bulbocavernosus reflex response latencies (Ertekin and Reel, 1976; Dick et al, 1974) may test the integrity of segmental circuits for erection.

Tests of vascular sufficiency are critical diagnostic procedures, considering that vascular disorders have been found in more than 60 percent of the patients evaluated at our sleep disorders center for impotence. Comparisons of brachial and penile arterial pressures (Gaskell, 1971; Abelson, 1975) as well as measurement of pulse volume and urethral temperature (Jevtich, 1981) in the flaccid penis, detect vascular insufficiency that can obstruct erection. If penile blood pressure in the right and left central arteries is much lower than brachial blood pressure, then vascular pathology is indicated. However, a false-normal Doppler penile reading may be obtained when accessory arteries that may exist or develop between the femoral and penile arteries compensate for occlusion in the major penile or epigastric arteries. These accessory arteries are incapable of circulating enough blood to the penis to allow full erection. When the proximal penile arteries are not completely patent, and the accessory arteries feed the penis, pressure applied to the femoral artery during the Doppler examination cuts off the blood flow in the accessory arteries and results in absent or diminished sound in the penile artery. A patient suffering from this vascular condition typically complains of pain in the buttocks accompanied by erectile competence of short duration (steal syndrome). Although in most patients arterial insufficiency is more likely to impair erection than venous pathology, a cavernosogram (Ginestié, 1980; Fitzpatrick, 1980) as well as an arteriogram (Michal et al., 1980) may also be necessary for differential diagnosis of vascular pathology.

We recently added penile temperature (Jevtich, 1981) as a test of circulatory sufficiency. Penile temperature measured via a thermometer inserted through the urethra to the base of the penis should be the same as the core body temperature measured deep under the back part of the tongue. A penile temperature at least 1 degree C lower than the body temperature may indicate circulatory problems.

Information from this series of procedures determines which systems will require more intensive examination during the NPT monitoring that follows or during the days between nocturnal monitorings.

Nocturnal penile tumescence is monitored on three consecutive nights as each patient sleeps in a private, environmentally controlled bedroom. Data from the first night, designated as an adjustment period to laboratory and monitoring conditions, are considered to be less reliable than data from subsequent nights, due to well-documented, atypical sleep patterns characteristic of the "first-night effect" (Rechtschaffen and Kales, 1968, Agnew et al., 1966; Jovanovíc, 1969). The second night provides the basic data on NPT patterns and the third night is reserved for special evaluations. The immediate objective is to determine whether NPT is normal, absent, or significantly diminished in comparison to normative data for the man's age group.

The patient reports to the sleep disorders center about 1½ hours before his customary bedtime to prepare for bed and complete a questionnaire about his activities that day, and for application of the monitoring devices. He retires and arises at his customary time and completes a questionnaire about the quantity and quality of his sleep upon arising. Bipolar, frontal, parietal, and occipital electrodes monitor electroencephalographic (EEG) activity and electrodes at the outer canthi of the eyes monitor electro-oculographic (EOG) activity. Two mercury-filled strain gauges sized to fit the patient monitor penile circumference changes; one encircles the base of the penis and the other is located just behind the glans. On at least one night (usually the third), the patient is awakened during his fullest erection for a photograph of his erect penis, an evaluation of degree and adequacy of erection, and an assessment of penile rigidity.

The NPT evaluation also includes more specific tests of neural, neuromuscular, and vascular function to confirm findings from the physical examination. An electrode in the perineal area detects bulbocavernosus-ischiocavernosus (BC-IC) activity, finger and penile electrodes monitor electrodermal activity (EDA), and a photoelectric transducer or a mercury strain gauge plethysmograph (Britt et al., 1971) over the dorsal penile artery measures penile pulse volume.

The pre-sleep questionnaire and nightly questioning by the technician and attending physician are designed to ensure that the patient is following instructions to avoid naps, excessive caffeine, alcohol, and nonessential drugs (especially psychoactive agents) during the evaluation period because they can disturb sleep and NPT patterns, thereby contaminating the polysomnographic data. However, the patient continues to take drugs required daily to determine whether these drugs might be contributing to his erectile impairment (Story, 1974). If NPT is impaired, the patient is re-evaluated under drug-free condtions.

The EEG and EOG evaluations serve as a validity check on the NPT data. Abnormal NPT recordings may actually reflect abnormal sleep rather than erectile dysfunction. The EEG-EOG recordings indicate whether sleep, especially REM sleep, is abnormally reduced or fragmented, or whether body movement artifacts are causing artificial pen excursions or penile circumference-change channels. The identification of the source of movement is especially important when a patient with spinal cord injury (Karacan et al., 1977a; 1978b) has muscle spasms in the lower trunk or legs because the erection is probably a segmental reflex rather than a normal erection. Our procedures for scoring EEG-EOG activity and NPT are described elsewhere (Rechtschaffen and Kales, 1968; Williams et al., 1974; Karacan et al., 1978c).

In normal men, increases in penile circumference represent the degree of erection. Since the base must expand 0.5 to 3 times more than the tip to allow vaginal penetration, polygraph tracings from both locations are essential. Inadequate tip expansion and rigidity often accompany impaired penile circulation or plaque while restricted base expansion often indicates a structural abnormality. In both of these pathological conditions, penile expansion is normal in one location, yet the abnormal discrepancies in expansion result in impotence. Therefore, several years ago we suggested that two gauges, one at the tip and the other at the base, should be used during NPT evaluation.

For the special NPT evaluation, the patient is awakened during an episode of tumescence estimated to be his maximum possible erection. The technician photographs the patient's erect penis to provide visual evidence of maximum erectile capacity, disease processes, or any structural defects. Meanwhile, both the patient and the technician estimate the degree of the patient's erection on a scale of 0 to 100 percent. The technician bases his estimate on such objective indicators as penile rigidity and the photograph. Therefore, if the patient's and technician's estimates are very discrepant, the patient may be unable to perceive the size of his erection accurately. Preliminary analyses suggest that impotent men with organically impaired NPT more often overestimate degree of erection than do men with psychologically impaired and better NPT. Further research is needed to determine whether this overestimation reflects a true perceptual failure, a self-image problem, or a deliberate misestimation for secondary gain. The results of the estimation procedure are consequently re-evaluated for possible psychological contributions to the patient's impotence.

Penile expansion does not always correlate with penile rigidity (which directly determines successful vaginal penetration) due to great individual differences among men. Therefore, we have developed a special device and procedure for evaluating this characteristic. After photographing the patient's penis, the technician presses the cap of the force-application device on the glans until the penis visibly bends. A constantin-foil, precision strain gauge, positioned along the dorsal midline of the penis, automatically detects ten-degree bending. The gauge measures buckling pressures between 1–1000 gm; 450 gm is the minimum buckling pressure at which satisfactory intercourse is possible.

Evaluation of spontaneous BC-IC activity during nocturnal erections—possibly reflecting autonomic activity—and of electrodermal activity during sleep uncovers neural deficits that may impair erectile capacity. Our finding (Karacan et al., 1978c) that spontaneous bursts of BC-IC muscle activity precede and accompany increases in penile circumference during

NPT episodes suggests that the muscles pump blood into the penis during erection. Bursts of muscle activity are absent or abnormal in some impotent men, suggesting that functional defects in these muscles may cause insufficient penile engorgement. Since the blood-pumping function is initiated in the higher CNS and most episodes of NPT occur during REM sleep, dissociation between REM and NPT in an impotent patient further confirms a CNS deficit.

We (Ware et al., 1980) have found that the pattern of electrodermal activity, which measures sympathetic activity during sleep, is also abnormal in some men with abnormal NPT. In normal men, sympathetic activity (EDA storms) diminishes during REM-related tumescence, but in some NPT-deficient patients activity continues during REM sleep and the period in which tumescence would normally occur. Perhaps this suggests that an imbalance between sympathetic and parasympathetic activity contributes to erectile dysfunction.

Monitoring penile pulse volume during episodes of NPT supplements the Doppler tests performed during the physical examination. The Doppler tests identify general vascular pathology and the pulse volume tests determine the extent to which such pathology contributes to erectile failure (Karacan and Salis, 1980). In normal men, pulse volume and penile circumference simultaneously increase when erection begins; there is little or no pulse volume response in some impotent men.

On one of the mornings during the three-day NPT evaluation, blood samples are drawn for hormone assays to evaluate the patient's endocrine status. Tests for testosterone (Rennie et al., 1939; Raboch and Starka, 1973; Lawrence and Swyer, 1974), prolactin (Thorner and Besser, 1977; Carter et al., 1978), luteinizing and follicle-stimulating hormone levels are particularly important because optimal levels may be necessary for adequate erectile functioning. As the final stage in the physiological evaluation, the drug history and drug levels in the urine are also examined; antihypertensive and psychoactive drugs especially appear to be associated with organogenic impotence (Story, 1974).

EVALUATION OF PSYCHOLOGICAL ETIOLOGY

If the results of the NPT evaluation and the supplementary physical examination and tests designate organogenic impotence, the patient is classified as having a physical disorder (Axis III) rather than a psychosexual disorder, ie, inhibited sexual excitement, or an Axis I mental disorder (eg, major depression). However, organic findings do not exclude the necessity of a thorough psychological evaluation; impotence is often of mixed etiology and emotional problems typically evolve from physical pathology, especially if the impotence is long-standing. Therefore, the ultimate objective of the psychological/psychiatric evaluation is differential diagnosis independent of the NPT evaluation. Unfortunately, there is no objective, systematic equivalent in the psychological evaluation to the NPT procedure. Relevant psychopathology can be identified from the psychiatric interview and psychological testing, but there is no definitive method for determining the extent of its contribution to impotence; identification of psychopathology does not necessarily signify psychological causes for the patient's erectile dysfunction. Therefore, psychogenic impotence essentially remains a default diagnosis, but positive evidence of psychological etiology is actively sought. In addition, since most impotent patients referred to our center are being considered by their urologist for implantation of a penile prosthesis (Scott, 1978), the psychiatric interview and psychological tests identify any psychiatric contraindications to the surgery.

The psychiatrist obtains a complete history; identifies any psychological, marital, or social problems; and assesses the patient's general mental status. To obtain the family and social histories, the patient and his spouse or sexual partner are each interviewed alone and then, if feasible, together. Possible indicators of psychogenic impotence are: (1) no long-term sexual relationships; (2) sudden onset in the absence of a traumatic condition or relevant medical complaint, especially when accompanied by marital discord; (3) reduced libido; (4) spontaneous occurrence of erections, such as upon awakening in the morning; and (5) wide variations in erectile capacity with different partners. There may also be a preponderance of such indicators as a premorbid history of premature ejaculation, homosexual activities, early sexual trauma, inordinate emotional closeness to his mother, and periods of adherence to rigid religious dictates. Beutler et al. (1978) more thoroughly describe psychonomic indicators for psychogenic impotence.

The other component of the psychological evaluation is the administration of a battery of written tests—Shipley's Institute of Living Scale (1940), the Minnesota Multiphasic Personality Inventory (MMPI) (Dahlstrom et al., 1972), the Loevinger Sentence Completion Test for Men (Loevinger and Wessler, 1978), the Profile of Mood States (McNair et al., 1971), the State-Trait Anxiety Inventory (Spielberger et al., 1970), Derogatis' Sexual Functioning Inventory (1976), the Locke-Wallace Marital Adjustment Scale (1959), and a special Reactions-to-Situations Scale (Schalling, 1977) designed to assess performance anxiety. These tests also assess degree of psychopathology, current mood, cognitive efficiency, interpersonal expectancies and needs, sexual disturbances, and defensive style.

Performance anxiety is an important diagnostic criterion—the APA's diagnostic manual (1980) stresses its involvement in inhibited sexual excitement, the psychogenic form of impotence. According to the APA, "Almost invariably a fear of failure and the development of a 'spectator' attitude (self monitoring) with extreme sensitivity to the sexual partner are present (in impotence). This may further impair performance and satisfaction and lead to secondary avoidance of sexual activity and impaired communication with the sexual partner." We (Karacan et al., 1980b) have recently found additional evidence that elevated state anxiety possibly accounts for psychogenic impotence. Masters and Johnson (1970) offer a comprehensive explanation of performance anxiety.

Defensive style, assessed via an MMPI index, also contributes to psychogenic impotence. Patients who emphasize internal defensive strategies—psychaesthenic, depressive, or obsessive defenses—are more likely to become psychogenically impotent than those who translate their conflicts into overt behaviors, as signified by hysterical, manic, paranoid, or psychopathic tendencies (Beutler et al., 1978). Correspondingly, the APA cites compulsive traits (internal defense) as well as any negative attitudes toward sexuality as predisposing factors to inhibited sexual excitement (1980).

Because of claims that the Derogatis Sexual Functioning Inventory (Derogatis, 1976; Karacan et al., 1980b) and certain indices from the MMPI (Beutler et al, 1975; 1976) can reliably discriminate between organogenic and psychogenic impotence, these two tests carry the most weight in the psychological evaluation.

Final psychological considerations when determining the extent of psychological etiology are evaluations of the patient's estimate of degree of erection when awakened during NPT monitoring. Men with organogenic impotence appear to overestimate their degree of erection. Asking the patient to explain how he arrived at his estimate is often helpful for distinguishing among deliberate misestimations, self-image problems, or perceptual difficulties. A patient may express disappointment or relief to visual evidence that he can or cannot have a full erection. Patients showing evidence of normal erectile capacity may be disappointed that there is no organic deficit to absolve them of a perceived "responsibility" for their impotence. This same finding may reassure other patients enough to improve their daytime sexual functioning.

ARRIVING AT A FINAL DIAGNOSIS

The final differential diagnosis represents the compiled, independent diagnoses of each team member—a urologist, an endocrinologist, a sleep researcher, a psychiatrist, and a psychologist, supplemented by any other specialists consulted. For example, a respiration and ear, nose and throat team may have been consulted to verify suspected sleep apnea, because this disorder may reflect generalized autonomic nervous system disturbance which could also impair erections. In determining whether impotence is primarily organogenic, psychogenic, or of mixed etiology, the NPT findings are emphasized. Absent or abnormally diminished NPT designates a high probability of organic involvement, with organic pathology more severe when there is no NPT. The cause of organogenic impotence is assessed by reviewing the various test and examination results. In at least ten percent of patients exhibiting impaired NPT and no gross psychopathology, our present series of physical, morphological, neural, vascular, endocrine, and psychological examinations are unable to determine the cause of impotence. This suggests that our current evaluation procedure may be omitting a critical test for some obscure contributor to erectile dysfunction. A better understanding of erectile impairment in such patients awaits: the more sophisticated study of the mechanisms of erectile failure; the search for exceptions, besides penile sensory defects, to the general rule that NPT is a reliable index of waking erectile capacity; the determination of the degree of vascular impairment required before erectile function is compromised; and a more comprehensive identification of drugs that affect erectile function. Crucial methodological modifications are needed to develop a more sensitive means of: (1) examining local and central autonomic system dysfunctions, (2) differentiating central from peripheral neural deficits, and (3) monitoring the interaction of psychological variables with physiological processes during sleep and sexual activity. Promising developments in sensitive transducer computer automation, as well as in understanding relevant neurotransmitters, are expected to improve our procedures for measuring indices of erectile dysfunction throughout the night.

ACKNOWLEDGMENT

The authors thank Ms Carol Howland of Baylor College of Medicine's Department of Psychiatry for editorial assistance in the preparation of this chapter.

REFERENCES

Abelson D: Diagnostic value of the penile pulse and blood pressure: A Doppler study of impotence in diabetics. *J Urol* 113:636–639, 1975

Agnew HW Jr, Webb WB, Williams RL: The first night effect: An EEG study of sleep. *Psychophysiology* 2:263–266, 1966.

American Psychiatric Association: *Diagnostic and Statistical Manual of Mental Disorders,* ed 3. Washington, DC, 1980, pp 275–279

Beutler LE, Karacan I, Anch AM, et al: MMPI and MIT discriminators of biogenic and psychogenic impotence. *J Consult Clin Psychol* 43:899–903, 1975

Beutler LE, Scott FB, Karacan I: Psychological screening of impotent men. *J Urol* 16:193–197, 1976

Beutler LE, Ware C, Karacan I: Psychological assessment of the sexually impotent male, in Williams RL, Karacan I (eds): *Sleep Disorders: Diagnosis and Treatment.* New York, John Wiley & Sons, 1978, pp 383–394.

Britt DB, Kemmerer WT, Robison JR: Penile blood flow determination by mercury strain gauge plethysmography. *Invest Urol* 8:673–678, 1971

Carter JN, Tyson JE, Tolis G, et al: Prolactin-secreting tumors and hypogonadism in 22 men. *N Engl J Med* 299: 847–852, 1978

Compere JS: Office recognition and management of erectile dysfunction. *Am Fam Physician* 17:186–190, 1978.

Cooper AJ: Factors in male sexual inadequacy: A review. *J Nerv Ment Dis* 149:337–359, 1969

Cooper AJ: The causes and management of impotence. *Postgrad Med J* 48:548–552, 1972.

Dahlstrom WG, Welsh GS, Dahlstrom LE: *An MMPI Handbook, vol. I: Clinical Interpretation.* Minneapolis, University of Minnesota, 1972.

Derogatis LR: Psychological assessment of sexual disorders, in Meyer JK (ed): *Clinical Management of Sexual Disorders.* Baltimore, Williams and Wilkins, 1976, pp 35–73

Derogatis LR, Meyer JK, Dupkin CN: Discrimination of organic versus psychogenic impotence with the DSFI. *J Sex Marital Ther* 2:229–240, 1976

Dick HC, Bradley WE, Scott FB, Timm GW: Pudendal sexual reflexes: Electrophysiologic investigations. *Urology* 3:376–379, 1974

Ertekin C, Reel F: Bulbocavernosus reflex in normal men and in patients with neurogenic bladder and/or impotence. *J Neurol Sci* 28:1–15, 1976

Finkel AL, Moyers TG, Tobenkin MI, Karg SJ: Sexual potency in aging males. Part 1. Frequency of coitus among clinical patients. *JAMA* 170:1391–1393, 1959.

Fisher C: Dreaming and sexuality, in Loewenstein RM, Newman LM, Schur M, Solnit AJ (eds): *Psychoanalysis—A General Psychology.* New York, International Universities Press, 1966, pp 537–569

Fisher C, Gross J, Zuch J: Cycle of penile erection synchronous with dreaming (REM) sleep. Preliminary report. *Arch Gen Psychiatry* 12:29–45, 1965

Fitzpatrick T: The venous drainage of the corpus cavernosum and spongiosum, in

Zorgniotti AW, Rossi G (eds): *Vasculogenic Impotence.* Springfield, Ill, Charles C Thomas, 1980, pp 181–184

Gaskell P: The importance of penile blood pressure in cases of impotence. *Can Med Assoc J* 105:1047–1051, 1971

Ginestié J-F: Cavernosography, in Zorgniotti AW, Rossi G (eds): *Vasculogenic Impotence.* Sprinfield, Ill, Charles C Thomas, 1980, pp 185–190

Halverson HM: Genital and sphincter behavior of the male infant. *J Genet Psychol* 56:95–136, 1940

Hastings DW: *Impotence and Frigidity.* Boston, Little, Brown & Co, 1963, p 45.

Hursch CF, Karacan I, Williams RL: Some characteristics of nocturnal penile tumescence in early middle-aged males. *Compr Psychiatry* 13:539–548, 1972

Jevtich MJ: Penile body temperature as screening test for penile arterial obstruction in impotence. *Urology* 17:132–135, 1981

Johnson J: Prognosis of disorders of sexual potency in the male. *J Psychosom Res* 9:195–200, 1965

Jovanović UJ: A new method of phallography (PhG). *Confin Neurol* 29:299–312, 1967

Jovanović UJ: Der effekt der ersten untersuchungsnacht auf die erektionen im Schlaf. *Psychother Psychosom* 17:295–308, 1969

Jovanović UF: *Sexuelle Reaktionen und Schlafperiodik bei Menschen. Ergebnisse experimenteller Untersuchungen.* Stuttgart, Ferdinand Enke Verlag, 1972

Kahn E, Fisher C: REM sleep and sexuality in the aged. *J Geriatr Psychiatry* 2:181–199, 1969

Kahn E, Fisher C: Some correlates of rapid eye movement sleep in the normal aged male. *J Nerv Ment Dis* 148:495–505, 1969

Karacan I: The effect of exciting presleep events on dream reporting and penile erections during sleep. New York, State University of New York, Downstate Medical Center, Department of Psychiatry, 1965 (doctoral dissertation)

Karacan I: The developmental aspect and the effect of certain clinical conditions upon penile erection during sleep. *Excerpta Medica International Congress Series,* No. 150. Proceedings of the IV World Congress of Psychiatry, Madrid, 1966, pp 2356–2359

Karacan I: A simple and inexpensive transducer for quantitative measurements of penile erection during sleep. *Behav Res Meth Instru* 1:251–252, 1969

Karacan I: Clinical value of nocturnal erection in the prognosis and diagnosis of impotence. *Med Asp Hum Sex* 4:27–34, 1970

Karacan I: Diagnosis of erectile impotence in diabetes mellitus. An objective and specific method. *Ann Intern Med* 92:334–337, 1980

Karacan I, Dervent A, Cunningham G, et al: Assessment of nocturnal penile tumescence as an objective method for evaluating sexual functioning in ESRD patients. *Dialysis Transplant* 7:872–876, 890, 1978a

Karacan I, Dervent A, Salis PJ, et al: Spinal cord injuries and NPT. *Sleep Res* 7:261, 1978b (abstract)

Karacan I, Dimitrijevic M, Lauber A, et al: Nocturnal penile tumescence (NPT) and sleep stages in patients with spinal cord injuries. *Sleep Res* 6:52, 1977a (abstract)

Karacan I, Goodenough DR, Shapiro A, Starker S: Erection cycle during sleep in relation to dream anxiety. *Arch Gen Psychiatry* 15:183–189, 1966

Karacan I, Hursch CJ, Williams RL: Some characteristics of nocturnal penile tumescence in elderly males. *J. Gerontol* 27:39–45, 1972a

Karacan I, Hursch CJ, Williams RL, Littell RC: Some characteristics of nocturnal penile tumescence during puberty. *Pediatr Res* 6:529–537, 1972b

Karacan I, Hursch CJ, Williams RL, Thornby JI: Some characteristics of nocturnal penile tumescence in young adults. *Arch Gen Psychiatry* 26:351–356, 1972c

Karacan I, Salis PJ: Diagnosis and treatment of erectile impotence. *Psychiatr Clin North Am* 3:97–111, 1980

Karacan I, Salis PJ, Thornby JI, Williams RL: The ontogeny of nocturnal penile tumescence. *Waking Sleeping* 1:27–44, 1976

Karacan I, Salis PJ, Williams RL: The role of the sleep laboratory in diagnosis and treatment of impotence, in Williams RL, Karacan I (eds): *Sleep Disorders: Diagnosis and Treatment.* New York, John Wiley & Sons, 1978c

Karacan I, Salis PJ, Ware JC, et al: Nocturnal penile tumescence and diagnosis in diabetic impotence. *Am J Psychiatry* 135:191–97, 1978d

Karacan I, Scott FB, Salis PJ, et al: Nocturnal erections, differential diagnosis of impotence, and diabetes. *Biol Psychiatry* 12:373–380, 1977b

Karacan I, Snyder S, Salis PJ, et al: Sexual dysfunction in male alcoholics and its objective evalution, in Fann WE, Karacan I, Pokorny AD, Williams RL (eds): *Phenomenology and Treatment of Alcoholism.* New York, Spectrum Publications, 1980a, 259–268

Karacan I, Ware JC, Dervent B, et al: Impotence and blood pressure in the flaccid penis: Relationship to nocturnal penile tumescence. *Sleep* 1:125–132, 1978e

Karacan I, Ware JC, Salis PJ, Goze N: Sexual arousal and activity: Effect on subsequent nocturnal penile tumescence patterns. *Sleep Res* 8:61, 1979 (abstract)

Karacan I, Ware JC, Salis PJ, Williams RL: Physiological and psychological characteristics of impotent men. *Sleep Res* 9:294, 1980b (abstract)

Karacan I, Williams RL, Salis PJ: The effect of sexual intercourse on sleep patterns and nocturnal penile erections. *Psychophysiology* 7:338–339, 1970 (abstract)

Karacan I, Williams RL, Thornby JI, Salis PJ: Sleep-related penile tumescence as a function of age. *Am J Psychiatry* 132:932–937, 1975

Kinsey AC, Pomeroy WB, Martin CE: *Sexual Behavior in the Human Male.* Philadelphia, W B Saunders Co, 1948, p 236

Keshin JG, Pinck BD: Impotentia. *NY State J Med* 49:269–272, 1949

Lawrence DM, Swyer GIM: Plasma testosterone and testosterone binding affinities in men with impotence, oligospermia, azoospermia, and hypogonadism. *Br Med J* 1:349–351, 1974

Levins, SB: Marital sexual dysfunction: Erectile dysfunction. *Ann Intern Med* 85:342–350, 1976

Locke HJ, Wallace KM: Short marital-adjustment and prediction tests: Their reliability and validity. *Marr Fam Living* 21:251–255, 1959

Loevinger J, Wessler R: *Measuring Ego Development, vol 1. Construction and Use of a Sentence Completion Test.* San Francisco, Jossey-Bass, 1978

Masters WH, Johnson VE: *Human Sexual Inadequacy.* Boston, Little Brown & Co, 1970, p. 183

McNair DM, Lorr M, Droppleman LF: *Manual for the Profile of Mood States.* San Diego, Educational and Industrial Testing Service, 1971

Michal V, Pospíchal J, Blažková J: Arteriography of the internal pudendal arteries and passive erection, in Zorgniotti AW, Rossi G (eds): *Vasculogenic Impotence.* Springfield, Ill, Charles C Thomas, 1980, pp 169–179

Moore C, Karacan I, Taylor A: Erectile dysfunction in Shy-Drager syndrome. *Sleep Res* 8:240, 1979 (abstract)

Ohlmeyer P, Brilmayer H: Periodische vorgänge im schlaf. II. Mitteilung. *Pfluegers Arch* 249:50–55, 1947

Ohlmeyer P, Brilmayer H,. Hüllstrung H: Periodische vorgänge im schlaf. *Pfluegers Arch* 248:559–560, 1944

Oswald I: *Sleep and Waking. Physiology and Psychology.* Amsterdam, Elsevier Publishing Co, 1962, p 142

Pearlman CK, Kobashi LI: Frequency of intercourse in men. *J Urol* 107:298–301, 1972

Pfeiffer E, Verwoerdt A, Davis GC: Sexual behavior in middle life. *Am J Psychiatry* 128:1262–1267, 1972

Raboch J: Two studies of male sex impotence. *J Sex Res* 6:181–187, 1970

Raboch J, Stárka L: Reported coital activity of men and levels of plasma testosterone. *Arch Sex Behav* 2:309–315, 1973

Rechtschaffen A, Kales A (eds): *A Manual of Standardized Terminology, Techniques and Scoring System for Sleep Stages of Human Subjects.* NIH Publication No. 204. US Government Printing Office, 1968

Rechtschaffen A, Verdone P: Amount of dreaming: Effect of incentive, adaptation to laboratory, and individual differences. *Percept Mot Skills* 19:947–958, 1964

Rennie TAC, Vest SA Jr, Howard JE: The use of testosterone proprionate in impotence: Clinical studies with male sex hormones (III). *South Med J* 32:1004–1007, 1939

Schalling D: The trait-situation interaction and the physiological correlates of behavior, in Magnusson D, Endler NS (eds): *Personality at the Crossroads: Current Issues in Interactional Psychology.* Hillsdale, NJ, Lawrence Erlbaum, 1977, pp 129–141

Scott FB: The surgical treatment of erectile impotence, in Williams RL, Karacan I (eds): *Sleep Disorders. Diagnosis and Treatment.* New York, John Wiley & Sons, 1978, pp 401–409

Shapiro A: Physiological characteristics of REM periods and related kinds of sleep. Presented at the Association for the Psychophysiological Study of Sleep, Palo Alto, March 1964

Shipley WC: A self-administering scale for measuring intellectual impairment and deterioration. *J Psychol* 9:371–377, 1940

Simpson SL: Impotence. *Br Med J* 1:692–697, 1950

Spielberger CD, Gorsuch RL, Lushene RE: *STAI Manual. For the State-Trait Anxiety Inventory ("Self-Evaluation Questionnaire")*. Palo Alto, Consulting Psychologists, 1970

Story NL: Sexual dysfunction resulting from drug side effects. *J Sex Res* 10:132–149, 1974

Strauss EB: Impotence from the psychiatric standpoint. *Br Med J* 1:697–699, 1950

Teoh JI, Lee M: Psychogenic impotence: Its aetiology, characteristics, and treatment by systematic desensitization. *Singapore Med J* 15:132–138, 1974

Thorner MO, Besser GM: Hyperprolactinaemia and gonadal function: Results of bromocriptine treatment, in Crosignani PG, Robyn C (eds): *Prolactin and Human Reproduction*. New York, Academic Press, 1977, pp 285–301

Verwoerdt A, Pfeiffer E, Wang H-S: Sexual behavior in senescence. Changes in sexual activity and interest of aging men and women. *J Geriatr Psychiatry* 2:163–180, 1968

Ware JC, Karacan I, Salis PJ, et al: Patterning of electrodermal activity during sleep: Relation to impotence. *Sleep Res* 9:296, 1980 (abstract)

Wershub LP: *Sexual Impotence in the Male*. Springfield, Ill, Charles C Thomas, 1959, pp 27, 29

Williams RL, Karacan I, Hursch CJ: *Electroencephalography (EEG) of Human Sleep: Clinical Applications*. New York, John Wiley & Sons, 1974

6

Diagnosis and Management of Gender Dysphoria

David W. Krueger

INTRODUCTION

Descriptive, dynamic, and developmental aspects of gender identity, as well as sexual role identity symptoms and syndromes, provide a basis for differentiating true transsexualism from pseudotranssexualism (patients who present with a self-diagnosis of transsexualism and a request for sex change surgery).

Two terms are important to distinguish. *Gender identity* is the internal representation of one's biological state, the sense of *maleness* (I am a man) or *femaleness* (I am a woman). Gender identity is established by age 2 or 3. The pathology of gender identity is transsexualism. *Sexual identity* is the identity of one's sex: masculinity or femininity. The characteristics and social role-appropriate behavior associated with one's gender are still components of sexual identity. The pathology of sexual identity manifests as paraphilias (sexual perversions). Sexual identity is established with and beyond the Oedipal period, i.e., beginning about age 3.

Far too little emphasis in the literature is placed on the diagnosis of the gender dysphoria syndrome of true transsexualism. Close scrutiny of the studies available regarding the transsexual syndrome, surgical selection criteria, and outcome reveals that patients with primary diagnoses other than true transsexualism are being diagnosed and surgically reassigned as transsexual. There is a large group of "pseudotranssexuals" who may present with a request for sex reassignment with a story compatible with Christine Jorgenson's or Renee Richards'. The patient with self-stated transsexualism presents with his own diagnosis and treatment program and has all the "correct" answers for the physician. The number of cases of lack of adjustment, regret, or worsening condition after sex change operations militates for a narrower definition of inclusion and exclusion criteria for the diagnosis of true transsexualism.

The purpose of this chapter is to present a review of work on diagnostic considerations of sexual gender and role identity symptoms and syndromes and to expand the consideration of pseudotranssexualism. Stress-induced regression in patients with certain psychopathology can eventuate in a request for sex change as a focus and a panacea. Additionally, patients with problems of identity (which may include sexual and gender identity) present with this request. The focus of transsexualism and belief in a surgical cure serves as an intrapsychic organizer for some of the patients who will be described.

EVALUATION PROCEDURES

The therapist's first task in evaluation is to establish a working alliance with the patient. This is crucial for the diagnostic assessment involving exploration of intimate and highly charged aspects of sexuality, fantasy, dreams, and relationships. The establishment of this rapport precedes the evaluation of highly charged material from the patient necessary for diagnostic consideration and for doing empathic work.

The initial work-up includes a complete physical examination, possible endocrinological and chromosomal studies, psychometric testing, and psychiatric evaluation. A standard exploratory psychiatric interview should include a special focus on family history, sexual history, current sexual behavior, psycho-social adjustment, gender role behavior, and mental status. Psychiatric evaluation should include not only material from the patient but also information from extensive interviews of the patient's family and other ancillary material as available, including longitudinal series of photographs or home movies of the patient as additional assessment information (Stoller, 1968).

Recognition and understanding of countertransference phenomenon is an important source of additional information about the patient. For example, the degree to which the patient is committed to and convincing about the social or sexual role may be revealed by the therapist's awareness of reactions to the patient, or by a slip in the use of a gender pronoun by the therapist. Even initial evaluations bring into focus the therapist's countertransferences, feelings about masculinity and femininity, and attitudes toward patients who want to change their anatomical sex.

It is important in the evaluation of this patient, as in all others, to consider the individual's total personality rather than to focus exclusively on the genuineness of the perceived gender disorder. The cry for help which is implicit in the transsexual request must be evaluated within a context which recognizes the patient as a complete human organism not limited to his presenting complaint (Kirkpatrick, 1920).

A brief evaluation is not appropriate. More extensive and exploratory diagnostic/therapeutic work involving a one to two year period of psychotherapy is prescribed for the patient who seems to meet the initial criteria for true transsexualism (Money and Ambinder, 1978; Newmann, 1970; Green et al,, 1966; Yalom et al., 1973; Stoller, 1973; Green et all., 1972). This period of psychotherapy explores the feasibility of reversing the patient's cross-gender orientation, provides diagnostic information regarding the potential for rehabilitation in social, vocational, economic, and emotional areas, and allows the therapist to assess the patient's developmental level and more closely observe areas of ego strength and psychopathology. The question of sex reassignment should be answered *last*, rather than in conjunction with other aspects of therapeutic planning done at the same time.

TRUE TRANSSEXUALS

Biologically male transsexuals

True transsexualism indicates a gender identity in biological males which is female both consciously and unconsciously, with a sexual role identity manifesting in femininity. This femininity is apparent from first gender behavior, around age 1, with no demonstrable masculine interests (Money and Ambinder, 1978). The conviction of being female and behaving femininely is *continuous*, as it is a gender identity and not an intermittent result of internal tension or a threat to masculinity. There is a pronounced wish to be a girl from first memory. Together with this history of wishing to be a girl is wanting his genitals changed to those of a female. There is no history of sexual arousal by cross-dressing, no history of being dressed in female clothes by someone else, and no history of sexual perversions (Money and Ambinder, 1978). The first request of the transsexual is to be rid of the offensive genitalia (not to have a vagina, but to be *rid of* male genitalia and give up male status). There is an eagerness to part with the penis. There is usually a rejection of homosexuality because it means acknowledgement of being male. Although the coital history may be heterosexual, homosexual, or bisexual, the usual underlying orientation is avoidant or asexual.

What happens developmentally to cause male transsexualism? The best evidence to date is that it begins in the first year of life, in the symbiotic union between mother and son. Stoller (1968) describes the mother as a woman with a strong bisexual component in her personality, who chose as her husband a man who is distant and passive. The mother finds the transsexual-to-be son beautiful and desires loving completeness with him. The two are profoundly close in sharing her femaleness; there is endless continuation of the merging of their bodies, as if they were one. The feminizing process continues by reinforcement of all that is not masculine, so this intense symbiosis is not disrupted. The feminizing process is uninterrupted by the father; the mother has insured that in her choice of husband.

The mother enjoys and encourages whatever keeps the child close to her, discouraging attempts to move away. The gender identity with the mother is complete and the discrepancy is then between gender identity and anatomical identity. By 3-5 years he talks of becoming a girl (which is an *identity* and a *role*) and a female (which is a *biological state*) when he grows up.

Because of inhibitions and internal splitting as defensive mechanisms in transsexualism, homosexuality as well as transvestism may be derivatives or steps toward the fully evolved manifestation of transsexualism. This makes differential diagnosis difficult; however, the conviction of transsexualism from early childhood and the degree of femininity and femaleness in the male patients are key elements in the assessment. The conviction of the patient that he is really a woman inside a male body should be scrutinized for its longevity, persistence, and conviction. This difficult and evolving clinical picture underscores the necessity for a one-to-two year trial period of evaluation and psychotherapy.

The transsexual's femininity may make him the object of teasing and he may attempt to hide the femininity. As he becomes unsuccessful at this and is, perhaps, friendless, an ensuing sadness and loneliness would lead to further isolation accompanied by poor object relatedness or developmental delay. The most consistent personality trend in male transsexuals is hysterical personality (Stoller, 1968; Finney et al., 1975).

Biologically Female Transsexuals

The biologically female transsexual believes herself to be a male both consciously and unconsciously. Female transsexuality is much less common and less is known about this condition. Female transsexuals live, dress, and work as men. They are similarly not using clothes as a fetishistic object, and do not have sexual relationships with men but are aroused only by women. They are not caricatures of "butch" homosexual women but are quietly passing undetected as men (Stoller, 1968). Their gender identity as a man both antedates and is much broader and more inclusive than the "penis envy" of the phallic-oedipal constellation in women.

The biologically female transsexual may be erotically attracted to females, just as the biologically male transsexual is erotically attracted to other males. While this may manifest as homosexuality, the breasts and absence of the penis are as loathsome as the presence of the penis is in the male. Breast fondling in the female transsexual, as well as penis fondling in the male transsexual, is not sexually exciting.

The relative rarity of female transsexualism may be related to the close contact of the female body of the mother in infancy, such that if pathological identifications occur it is more likely in the male's cross-gender identification with the mother (Stoller, 1968). This task of resolving cross-gender identification with the early primary love object is not a problem of females.

Indeed, a consistent finding and possible cause of transsexualism in the biological female is a very early severance in the relationship with the mother, followed by the assumption of the primary caretaking role by an overly close and solicitous father who may encourage toughness and aggression.

PSEUDOTRANSSEXUALISM: SYMPTOMS AND SYNDROMES

True transsexualism as an entity independent of other mental disorders must be firmly established. True transsexualism must be clearly distinguished from the transsexual *symptom* or transsexual *desires*, which may represent a regressive defense against anxiety crystallized by intense emotional stress. Other forms of psychopathology in patients resulting in a chronic miserable life circumstance may result in a patient seeking "transformation." The desire for sexual reassignment may be transitory, the manifestation of a concretized need for total or global change, and thus based on a basic pathology other than true transsexualism (Newman and Stoller, 1974).

The following discussion is a classification of the types of "pseudotranssexuals" and the pathological mechanism in each resulting in the transsexual wish.

Transvestism

The transvestite is dependent on fetishistic imagery or behavior involving women's clothing for sexual arousal and orgasm. Gender identity is male; sexual role identity is masculine. These patients are not effeminate; maleness and masculinity are well developed. The transvestite's earliest conviction is that he is a male and that his penis has much importance. The distinguishing feature of this syndrome is that putting on clothes of the opposite sex produces unquestioned genital excitement (Stoller, 1978). A history of fetishism, even if brief, is an important diagnostic indicant in individuals requesting sex change surgery, as it represents a positive attachment to the penis, supporting a diagnosis of homosexuality or transvestism rather than transsexualism (Newman and Stoller, 1974).

Masculinity therefore emerges in the transvestite (as in the homosexual, but unlike the transsexual), yet masculinity is shaped by the mother or an important and dominant female. The transvestite is dependent upon cross-dressing for the relief of an insistent and overpowering tension. Masculinity is protected by regressing to earlier identification with the mother, and the rituals of perversion serve the function of undoing separation (Stoller, 1978). An essential element in the paraphilias (homosexuality, transvestism, and other sexual identity disorders) is a regression to masculinity, i.e., masculinity was present at some time (Bak, 1968). Masculinity has never been present with a true transsexual.

The transvestite may occasionally have transsexual fantasies, especially at times of severe stress when cross-dressing does not relieve the overwhelming tension emanating from some threat to his masculinity. At these times regression may occur to a more primitive fantasy in a reparative effort of symbiotic union with the mother; this merger with the mother is identified by the patient as transsexual and there is a wish to surgically complete this union (Person and Ovesey, 1978).

Meyer (1974) has described a population of aging tranvestites who seek consultation in middle life for sex reassignment, characteristically because of depression and suicidal ideation, with the patients often in depersonalized or dissociated states. These patients present requesting change at a time when cross-dressing loses its capacity for sexual arousal.

Effeminate Homosexuality

The homosexual's gender identity is male and sexual role identity is effeminate, infused to varying degrees with mimicry, hatred, and fear. There is evidence of this effeminate behavior early in childhood. Homosexual relations focus on his penis, antithetical to transsexuals. There is erotic attachment to men. Male genitalia are prized and there is usually no seeking to change male status.

There is no compulsion to wear women's clothes as in transvestism, but occasionally the homosexual may do so for the purpose of attracting other men; however, there is no fetishistic arousal per se. The homosexual does not have a compulsion to cross-dress or to be a woman; his genitals are an integral part of his sexual identity, involving the derivation of erotic pleasure from receiving or providing satisfaction with another male.

Homosexuality is not a homogeneous condition in which a clear-cut diagnostic category exists of the same syndrome and etiology. Homosexuality must be differentiated as a sympton from a syndrome, with consideration of stress, conflict, and regression. The male homosexual, like the transvestite and unlike the transsexual, has developed masculinity in childhood which is threatened by either or both parents, making the continuing development of comfortable masculinity difficult and filled with conflict. Emerging masculinity is shaped by the mother in an overprotective environment which forbids "distasteful behavior": rough, penetrating, physically assertive, dirty, or heterosexual.

Transvestism and homosexuality are basically conflictual developmental issues of psychosexual, separation-individuation, and/narcissistic lines with regression along one or more lines at times resulting in a transsexual request. Table 1 outlines qualities which differentiate these developmental conflicts from transsexualism.

Borderline and Narcissistic Personality Disorders

In the borderline personality, a stable sense of self and identity solidification does not emerge. The failure to adequately negotiate and resolve these issues of separation-individuation results in identity diffusion and inadequate sense of self. The synthesis and integration of different isolated self-representations which produce identity (Jacobsen, 1964)

TABLE 1. DIFFERENTIATING QUALITIES OF TRANSSEXUALISM AND PSEUDOTRANSSEXUALISM

	Gender Identity	Sexual Role Identity	Sexual Fantasy Life	Sexual Behavior	Social Role
Transsexualism	Female (conscious and unconscious)	Feminine	Pronounced wish to be a girl, to be rid of offensive genitalia	Asexual; abhorrence of male genitalia. No sexual arousal by cross-dressing (interest in *outer* garments). No history of fetishism	In early adulthood may make one last effort to be masculine; when this fails, depression ensues
Transvestism	Male	Masculine	Dependent on fetishistic imagery or behavior for sexual arousal	Heterosexual	Lives and works as a man. Usually married and a father
Effeminate Homosexuality	Male	Effeminate	Erotic attraction to men	Homosexual, no abhorrence of genitalia	No drive to be a woman, yet has effeminate interests and pursuits that *mimic* women

does not occur. Gender issues may be manifestations of this incomplete and unstable sense of self and identity in the following way. Diffusion may be crystallized into a false self (an identity of the opposite sex) in an attempt to avoid abandonment depression in a borderline personality or in an attempt to focus a fragmented self in narcissistic patients. The sex and gender issues may be seized upon as a unifying focus for the various facets of identity diffusion. The exursion into an "as if" orientation may merely represent one of the more recent attempts at resolving basic developmental conflicts. A patient's sense of identity at times of fragmentation may achieve a separate autonomy in the form of roles. A *transsexual role* is possible in some patients. This regression fragments the patient's fragile sense of identity, including gender identity, into primitive fusions of self and object, notably fusion with and introjection of the mother. This may culminate in a conviction of transsexualism resulting in a request for surgical operation. The sex change would then represent a union and symbiotic fusion with the mother—the ultimate bond which is longed for, a longing driven by separation anxiety.

Sexual behavior of the borderline personality is characterized descriptively as polymorphous perverse. This range of pathological sexuality is a manifestation of disordered internalized object relationships. Other characteristics of the lower level borderline personality disorder are evident when a longitudinal descriptive and dynamic diagnosis is made.

In the person with narcissistic pathology, one basis of sexual perversions may lie in the child's experiences of self-objects whose empathic and mirroring responses would not be consistently or accurately attained in order for a healthy development and consolidation of the self to occur (Kohut, 1978). Having failed to experience stimulating responses from others, he then attempts to stimulate isolated body zones via isolated drives (fetishism), attempts to look for a response from the idealized self-object (exhibitionism), or merges with an idealized maternal imago (pseudotranssexualism). Perverse activity is similar to addiction, with craving for self-enhancing and validating experiences in the narcissistically vulnerable individual.

Schizoid and Avoidant Character Disorders

The diagnostic groups of schizoid and avoidant personalities perceive the need for a major change in their lives if they are to have satisfying and meaningful relationships. These patients may detail a history of unhappiness in interpersonal relationships, finding it difficult to become close to anyone in particular. Trying sexual relationships with both men and women, these patients found nothing really satisfactory, precluding the enjoyment of sex. There is often acute sensitivity and susceptability to rejection in relationships, and the frequent, sometimes accurate, fear of being found unattractive by the opposite sex. A history of shyness as a child and an excessive fear of social situations may be present. Masturbatory fantasies and orgastic experiences are austere and somewhat divested of object relatedness.

The need for change may be concretized as the need to change the external sex and try the other one. The propensity is to idealize the opposite sex and unconsciously hope that by "splitting," good and bad objects can be separately maintained. The sex change request then would be for the removal (absolute projection) of those characteristics seen as "bad" or which identify him with the hated and depreciated parent of the same sex.

In extended evaluation psychotherapy the transsexual request is seen to be a combination of withdrawal from object relationships and an artificial attempt at social adaptation. This withdrawal is in contrast to the true transsexual who may attempt to hide his femininity and secondarily experiences isolation and loneliness due to not "fitting in."

Psychotic Disorders

Patients with psychotic disorders often have gross disturbances of sexual role identity and gender identity, with hallucinations or delusions of body changes as if their anatomy were that of the opposite sex. Here too, the focus of transsexual desires may become an overdetermined and insistent one. Upon closer scrutiny of the patient's total psychiatric picture, transsexualism is seen to be a representation of ego disintegration. This may manifest as feelings that one is losing the attributes of a sex or gender which he prizes, and a dissolving of the sense of self and its representation of identity, including gender identity. In reintegration, delusions or hallucinations of being the opposite sex serve a reparative function to organize the patient's disintegration in a magical way.

Intersexuality

Intersexuality refers to those patients with anatomical, hormonal, or physiological aspects of one or both anatomical sexes. Included are chromosomal disorders (Turner's and Klinefelter's syndromes), pseudohermaphroditism, ova-testes, adrenogenital syndrome, hypogonadism, gonadal disgenesis. Temporal lobe epilepsy may also present as a transvestite or transsexual disorder while being physiologically based (Blumer, 1969). These disorders emphasize the importance of an initial physical, endocrinologic, and chromosomal examination as a first step.

DISCUSSION

A desire for sex change of relatively recent onset may represent a perceived magical escape from a particular life crisis, chronic discomfort, or crisis in sexual identity (Kirkpatrick, 1920; Newman, 1974). As the crisis precipitating the desire for "change" passes, so usually does the wish for sexual reassignment, unless it is reinforced by the therapist. The desire may have been crystallized externally—such as by hearing interviews or accounts of transsexuals whose lives have undergone significant change due to reassignment surgery—or internally—by the loss of an important object (e.g., Mother) and the attempt to fuse with that object. Chronic unhappiness and discomfort may particularly manifest in a sexual context in those personalities already having significant latent cross-gender identification; problems may then be attributed to the gender role of the patient. Transsexual themes resulting in request for surgery may be seen as a panacea for this discomfort, an attempt to split off the "bad" self and become an idealized "good" self.

Morgan (1978) has aptly pointed out that "any person applying for sex reassignment surgery has a serious problem." Differentiating gender dysphoria syndrome from symptom, making a developmental, dynamic, and descriptive diagnosis, and understanding the precipitants for presentation at a particular time are all important aspects of evaluation.

Available evidence suggests that the true transsexual does not benefit from psychotherapy regarding the transsexual syndrome reversal per se (Newman, 1970; Baker and Green, 1970), but psychotherapy is essential for several reasons. A minimum period of one to two years is important for the true transsexual in differentiating the intensity, persistence, and the strength of his drive for sex change surgery. The stability of this drive is unique to the transsexual. Psychotherapy can serve as both an important diagnostic tool and a support to the true transsexual in adjusting to his situation with or without sex reassignment. Sexual reassignment represents a loss and a change, the like of which the patient has never seen and which will affect his life unpredictably; similarly, the irreversibility of genital change and the impossibility of surgical reassignment all involve losses and concomitant readjustment. Psychotherapy may allow us to study the dynamics and etiology of true transsexualism as well as the precipitants of stress which induce the particular types of regressions manifesting in a request for sex reassignment surgery. Additionally, the flexibility to explore his psyche in therapy would be a good prognostic indicator of the patient's ability to successfully cross genders, social and sexual roles, and identities.

Core gender identity can be viewed as a continuum, never all-or-nothing. The efforts to develop objective criteria and standardization of some diagnostic procedures, along with validation by family and professional third parties, will hopefully make scientific data collection more clinically useful to the patient (Mackenzie, 1978). There is evidence that the patients selected precisely for the most severe identity problems, whose problems are more specific and circumscribed to gender identity dysphoria (ie, specific diagnostic inclusion and exclusion criteria), do better with sex reassignment surgery (Money and Ambinder, 1978; Walinder et al., 1978; Benjamin, 1966; Fisk, 1978).

The emphasis on diagnosis is for more appropriate treatment of patients facing an irreversible and profound surgical maneuver, to refine our diagnostic precision in our future work, and to understand etiological factors more fully. An insistent and abiding detailed follow-up of cases will help us achieve precision regarding the specific inclusion and exclusion criteria for true transsexualism. Further refinement of criteria from the best results may help us to understand etiological factors more fully and aid us in studying the related yet parallel developmental issues of object relationships, sense of self, and psychosexual and gender development.

REFERENCES

Bak R: The phallic woman: The ubiquitous fantasy in perversion. *Psychoanal Study Child* 23: 15–36, 1968

Baker H, Green R: Treatment of transsexualism. *Curr Psychiat Ther* 10: 88–89, 1970

Benjamin H: *The Transsexual Phenomenon*. New York, The Julian Press Inc, 1966

Blumer D: Transsexualism, sexual dysfunction, and temporal lobe disorder, in Green R, Money J (eds): *Transsexualism and Sex Reassignment*. Baltimore, Johns Hopkins Press, 1969

Finney J, Brandsma J, Rondow M, Lemaistre G: A study of transsexuals seeking gender assignment. *Am J Psychiat* 132: 962–964, 1975

Fisk N: Five spectacular results. *Arch Sex Behav* 7: 351–369, 1978

Green R, Newman L, Stoller R: Treatment of boyhood transsexualism. *Arch Gen Psychiatry* 26: 213–217, 1972

Green R, Stoller R, MacAndrews C: Attitudes toward sex transformation procedures. *Arch Gen Psychiatry* 15: 178–182, 1966

Jacobson E: *The Self and the Object World.* New York, International Universities Press, 1964

Kirkpatrick M, Friedmann C: Treatment of request for sex change surgery with psychotherapy. *Am J Psychiatry* 133: 1194–1196, 1976

Kohut H: A note on female sexuality, in Ornstein P (ed): *The Search for the Self: Selected Writings of Hering Hohut: 1950–1978,* vol 2. New York, International Universities Press, 1978

MacKenzie K: Gender dysphoria syndrome: Towards standardized diagnostic criteria. *Arch Sex Behav* 7: 251–262, 1978

Meyer J: Clinical variance among applicants for sex reassignment. *Arch Sex Behav* 3: 527–558, 1974

Money J, Ambinder R: Transsexualism: Indications for surgical treatment, in Brady J, Brodie H (eds): *Controversy in Psychiatry* Philadelphia, W. B. Saunders, 1978

Morgan A: Psychotherapy for transsexual candidates screened out of surgery. *Arch Sex Behav* 7: 272–283, 1978

Newman L: Transsexualism in adolescents: Problems in evaluation and treatment. *Arch Gen Psychiatry* 23: 112–121, 1970

Newman L, Stoller R: Non-transsexual men who seek reassignment. *Am J Psychiatry* 131: 437–441, 1974

Person E, Ovesey L: Transvestism: New perspectives. *J Am Acad Psychoanal* 6: 301–323, 1978

Stoller R: *Sex and Gender,* vol 1. New York, Jason Arronson, 1968

Stoller RJ: Male transsexualism: Uneasiness. *Am J Psychiatry* 130: 536–539, 1973

Stoller R: Boyhood gender aberrations: Treatment issues. *J Am Psychoanal Assoc* 26: 541–558, 1978

Walinder J, Lundstrom B, Thuwe I: Prognostic factors in the assignment of male transsexuals for sex reassignment. *Br J Psychiatry* 132: 16–20, 1978

Yalom I, Green R, Fisk N: Prenatal exposure to female hormones. *Arch Gen Psychiatry* 28: 554–561, 1973

7

Sexual Adjustment in the Physically Handicapped

Lauro S. Halstead

INTRODUCTION

Historical Information

One of the most important developments in health care over the past two decades has been the increased interest in and emphasis on sexual health. This has been true for able-bodied and disabled persons alike. Rehabilitation medicine has played an important role in helping to increase awareness of sexual problems and rights, especially for individuals with physical impairments. As a result of this increased interest in sexuality, there have been numerous studies which have uniformly confirmed that persons with a wide range of disabilities retain a strong interest in remaining sexually active and fulfilled.

One of the ironies of this increased emphasis on sexuality is that the available resources and information on sexual function and dysfunction remain inadequate to meet the demand. However, it is also clear that many of the expectations and needs of disabled persons with questions and problems in the area of sexuality can be met by persons without specialized training or skill in sexual matters. Frequently, an expression of interest, an understanding and nonjudgmental attitude, and straightforward candid information about sexual function are all that is needed to sanction a patient's desire to resume sexual activity or attempt various sexual options or alternative modes of sexual expression.

Definitions

It is important to keep in mind the difference between "sex" and "sexuality." Sex is a limited term which refers to genital activity. By contrast, sexuality is a much broader term which refers to many facets of a person's self-concept and identity. Major components included in the term sexuality are (a) psychological considerations which deal with self-concept, (b) social-sexual elements which refer to how we relate to other persons of the opposite and the same sex, and (c) behavioral aspects which deal with specific sexual activities. A partial list of these activities includes genital and nongenital physical contact, self-pleasuring and pleasuring of a sexual partner, intimacy, caring, and verbal and nonverbal communication.

BARRIERS TO INCLUDING SEXUALITY AS PART OF HEALTH CARE

Attitudes

There are a number of barriers which impede the delivery of effective sexual health care to disabled persons. Two of the most common are negative attitudes about sexuality and lack of information about normal sexual function and changes in the presence of a specific disease process. Negative attitudes and lack of information lead, in turn, to the creation of a third barrier—myths. In part, these myths imply that disabled persons are uninterested in sex, do not function normally anyway, and might hurt themselves in some way. Such myths help perpetuate negative attitudes and misinformation. Of all these barriers, however, negative attitudes are the most formidable obstacle because they tend to determine what we think, say, and do as professionals and patients.

Physician   Because sexuality is such a personal and intimate matter, physicians, along with everyone else, have strong feelings and emotions with respect to their own sexuality as well as that of others. No area of medicine creates more anxiety and apprehension than sexuality; this explains in part why this area has been neglected for so long, and why it is so difficult for most physicians to deal with sexual problems. As a consequence of those strong attitudes, it is easy for the physician to project any inhibitions, anxieties, or prejudices he might have onto patients. In addition, his own sense of discomfort acts as a barrier or inhibitor to taking the initiative in discussing possible areas of sexual dysfunction or dissatisfaction. Being aware of these barriers and potential biases is an important first step in opening a productive dialogue with patients.

For most physicians, becoming comfortable with the topic of sexuality and developing a facility in the area requires training and practice. As in many other areas of health care delivery, one's own personal experiences or study are not sufficient. Many sex educators and counselors believe that one of the most effective techniques in helping people reevaluate their personal and professional feelings regarding sexuality has been the Sexual Attitude Reassessment (SAR) Program developed by the National Sex and Drug Forum in San Francisco and now available in many centers throughout the United States. Variations of this program are also sponsored by churches and other community groups (See Appendix for a list of SAR programs and other resources in the area of sexuality and disability).

Patient As with the physician, patient attitudes about sexuality are determined by upbringing, moral and ethical values, personal experience, and level of satisfaction. In addition, attitudes may be seriously altered by their disability as well. This is especially true in persons with altered neuromuscular development and control or those who have sustained a significant alteration in physical appearance or function.

Society This refers to the influences all of us experience during our formative years from family, friends, schools, church, and other social institutions. It also relates to legal and moral sanctions which permit or condemn various sexual practices. And finally, it refers to regulations and policies within health care institutions such as hospitals, extended care facilities, and nursing homes, which either inhibit or facilitate various kinds of sexual behaviors and interactions. As a practical example, many of these influences play a role in determining whether a hospital will provide a privacy room for its patients, where they can be undisturbed and on their own to do whatever they choose.

Value Clarification

One way for an individual to clarify his values with regard to various sexual behaviors is to identify which kinds of activities he feels comfortable with and which activities cause mild or strong discomfort. Figure 1 shows Sexual Attitude Scales used at the Sexual Attitude Reassessment Program in Houston, Texas. Participants are asked in the context of privacy and confidentiality to indicate how they feel about the sexual activities listed.

Sexual Attitude Scales

Instructions: Please indicate how you feel about these specific activities using the following alternative responses.

1 = I feel *great* about it
2 = I feel *comfortable* about it
3 = I feel *indifferent* about it
4 = I feel *uncomfortable* about it
5 = I feel *repulsed* about it

Circle the number of your response for each activity in the space provided.
(EXAMPLE: 1 2 3 4 5) Please answer all questions.

1. Using erotica (erotic literature, pictures, films, live sex shows, etc) to stimulate sexual arousal:

   1 2 3 4 5   for yourself   1 2 3 4 5   for other adults

2. Fantasy as a sexual stimulant in private masturbation:

   1 2 3 4 5   for yourself   1 2 3 4 5   for other adults

3. Mutual masturbation with someone of the opposite sex:

   1 2 3 4 5   for yourself   1 2 3 4 5   for other adults

4. Mutual masturbation with someone of the same sex:

1   2   3   4   5   for yourself   1   2   3   4   5   for other adults

5. Sexual intercourse with someone of the opposite sex:

1   2   3   4   5   for yourself   1   2   3   4   5   for other adults

6. Oral-genital stimulation with someone of the opposite sex:

1   2   3   4   5   for yourself   1   2   3   4   5   for other adults

7. Oral-genital stimulation with someone of the same sex:

1   2   3   4   5   for yourself   1   2   3   4   5   for other adults

8. Engaging in sex with your partner in the presence of others:

1   2   3   4   5   for yourself   1   2   3   4   5   for other adults

9. Three or more people engaging in intercourse and other sexual activity together:

1   2   3   4   5   for yourself   1   2   3   4   5   for other adults

FIG. 1. Sexual Attitude Reassessment (SAR) Workshop

Another way of clarifying your own sexual values is to take one of those activities—for example, masturbation—and consider for a moment how you feel about that activity in a variety of contexts. For example, how you feel about masturbation when performed by your spouse or sexual partner, when performed by your teenaged daughter, by your mother, by a patient with a stroke, or by a patient with mental retardation. Extensions of this might include such questions as, "How do you feel about patients masturbating while they are in the hospital?" "Does it make a difference whether it takes place in a private room, a semi-private room, or a ward?" "How do you feel about a patient's spouse or sexual partner masturbating the patient if the patient cannot do it for himself?" "How do you feel about masturbation being provided by a member of the hospital staff?" "Is this professional and ethical?" "Is this therapeutically justifiable for a patient who is unable to do it for himself?" "Should a hospital provide a privacy room for a patient or patients to perform sexual activities?"

These questions are intentionally confined to the activity of masturbation; however, similar questions could also be raised about a number of other sexual behaviors. How you feel about these questions and what you would say and do about them on behalf of your patients reflect your own sexual attitudes and beliefs. If some of these questions make you feel uncomfortable, it may be of interest to explore why. It may also be useful to ask yourself if your discomfort interferes with your providing full and competent health care to your clients.

Information

Sexual Response Cycle in Able-Bodied Persons   The sexual response cycles for able-bodied males and females are shown in Figures 2 and 3. Although there is a broad range of sexual responses, these figures show four phases which are common to both sexes. These include excitement, plateau, orgasm, and resolution. In addition to these general phases, Masters and Johnson (1966) have identified discrete physiologic and anatomic responses for various organ systems.

Sexual Response Cycle in Disabled Persons   In contrast to our knowledge about the sexual response cycle in able-bodied persons, much less is known concerning similar responses in persons with various disabilities. As noted previously, this lack of information often makes it difficult for the counseling physician to provide specific information which could be helpful in both diagnosis and treatment.

Examples of the physiologic responses during the sexual response cy-

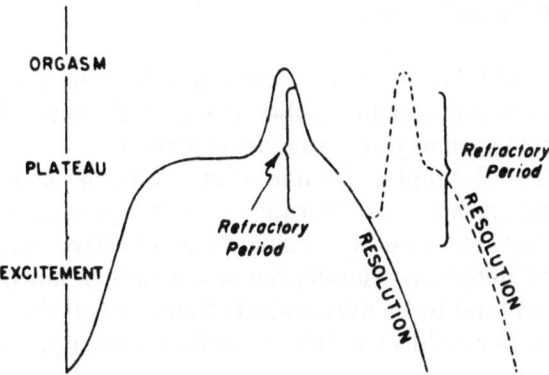

FIG. 2. Sexual response cycle in able-bodied men (from Masters and Johnson, 1966).

cles in males and females with spinal cord injury are shown in Tables 1 and 2. As can be seen, information with regard to specific responses of the female during the sexual response cycle is incomplete. Similar gaps are also present for many other disability groups either because they have not yet been investigated or because the techniques which permit adequate assessment have not been developed. It is hoped that with the increased interest in helping patients become as sexually active as they would like, more information will become available; thus, physicians will be better able to provide appropriate counseling and therapeutic intervention.

CLASSIFICATION OF DISABILITIES

There are three major factors to consider in approaching patients with physical disabilities. These include time of onset, stability of the lesion, and visibility of the impairment to others. Although there are frequently many features in common, no two disabled persons are alike. They combine their sexual attitudes and experiences and their disability experiences in ways which are obviously different and unique. For this reason, the following classification of disabilities is helpful in approaching individual patients with specific sexual problems.

Disabilities Prior to Puberty

Stable Conditions such as congenital loss of limbs or sight or traumatic amputations before puberty will significantly alter normal psychological and psychosocial sexual development.

Progressive Examples include cystic fibrosis and muscular dystrophy. Through improved therapeutic techniques, many of these children are living longer and becoming sexually active. Again, the specific disability will determine the degree of restriction; however, in general, these children tend to be overprotected and denied the experiences and information other children obtain regarding sexuality.

Post-Puberty Disabilities

Stable This category includes spinal cord injury, traumatic amputation, coronary heart disease, and stroke, to name a few. A major consideration in these disorders is whether they are conspicuous to other members of society. Although there may be a psychological stigma in each instance, the alteration in body image experienced by a stroke victim or a patient with a spinal cord injury plays a major role in how they see themselves as sexual persons and potential sexual partners.

Progressive This category includes such disorders as multiple sclerosis, arthritis, progressive blindness, etc. As mentioned before, disorders which are visible to others will have a different impact on a per-

TABLE 1. COMPARISON OF SEXUAL RESPONSE CYCLES IN ABLE-BODIED AND SPINAL CORD INJURED (SCI) MALES

	Able-Bodied Male	SCI Male
Penis	erects	frequent
Skin or Scrotum	tenses	frequent
Testes	elevate in scrotum	frequent
Emission	yes	infrequent
Ejaculation	yes	infrequent

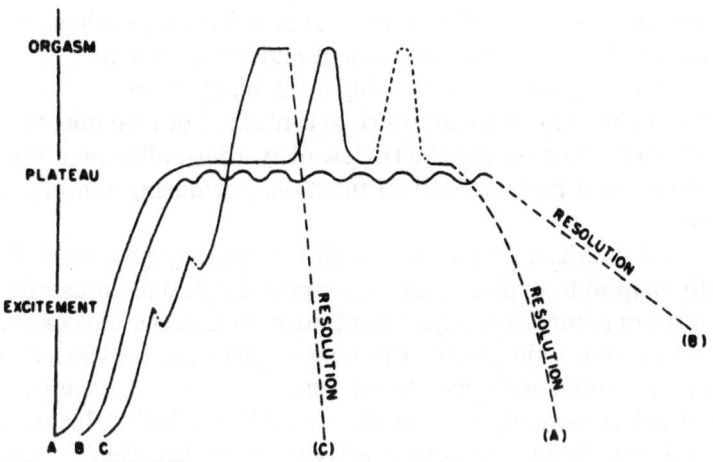

FIG. 3. Sexual response cycle in able-bodied women (from Masters and Johnson, 1966).

son's sexual self-concept and social/sexual relations than a disability which is not visible.

ASSESSMENT OF SEXUAL PROBLEMS

History

A thorough history of sexual function and enjoyment, taken with tact and candor, can be therapeutic as well as diagnostic. For many patients, your sexual history may be the first any physician has ever taken. The simple fact that you are sufficiently concerned to ask questions can relieve the patient's sense of anxiety, isolation, and frustration.

When taking a sexual history, it may be helpful to bear in mind that studies have shown that the level of sexual activity varies from disability to disability, and will obviously depend upon the age of the individual patient. In one study of 640 disabled and able-bodied persons for the behaviors of masturbation, intercourse, and oral/genital activity, the level of sexual activity for disabled adults was approximately 20–30 percent less than that of persons without disabilities. By contrast, in the same study, the level of satisfaction (approximately 40 percent) was surprisingly similar for both groups. Reasons for dissatisfaction were fairly similar and included lack of partners, communication problems, and lack of interest on the part of the respondent and/or the partner.

Some practical guidelines for taking a sex history are:

1. Take the history in an appropriate context. For example, the sexual history may be taken during the review of systems, after inquiring about genitourinary and gastrointestinal functions, or during the physical examination.

2. Be systematic. For patients with a relatively new disability it is especially helpful to explore three time periods: sexual adjustment prior to the onset of symptoms, adjustment during exacerbations or complications, and present adjustment. Previous adjustment provides a good insight into potential outcome. Some questions to ask include: "Is the patient as active sexually as he or she would like to be?" "Has the disability caused any change in sexual activity or satisfaction?" "Are there reasons for decreased satisfaction?" "When did these begin?"

3. Explore feelings of loss. Even in mild cases, most persons with physical limitations feel they have experienced a loss, which affects the way they view themselves. Questions to ask the patient include: "What do you feel you have lost?" "Has it changed your self-image?" "Do you feel less masculine or less feminine?"

4. Set realistic goals. As a result of the history, the physician should gain a general idea of how knowledgeable the person is about sexual activity and function, the level of satisfaction and any areas of dissatisfac-

TABLE 2. COMPARISON OF SEXUAL RESPONSE CYCLES IN ABLE-BODIED AND SPINAL CORD INJURED (SCI) FEMALES

	Able-Bodied Female	SCI Female
Wall of Vagina	moistens	———
Clitoris	swells	swells
Labia	swells and opens	swells
Uterus	contracts	———
Inner ⅔ of Vagina	expands	———
Outer ⅓ of Vagina	contracts	———

tion or dysfunction, an overview of the patient's range of sexual behaviors and his/her willingness to explore new options.

Physical Examination

There are a number of areas of the physical examination which require special emphasis and which can provide helpful information in making either a diagnosis or therapeutic suggestion. These include:

1. Strength, endurance, coordination, and mobility. Can the patient control his movements to the extent that he can assume an active role in lovemaking, or will he need to be more passive? What is the extent or limitation of arm and hand dexterity? If a male patient is having difficulty with erections, assessment of wrist, hand, and finger function is important, as these can be used effectively to provide sexual stimulation and gratification for the partner.

2. Sensation. In patients with sensory deficits, it is helpful to identify areas of preserved or normal sensation. Many patients with sensory deficits report shifting of erogenous zones away from the genitals to other areas such as the axilla, neck, etc. Even areas of diminished sensation, especially around the genitals or anus, can become highly erotic and play an important role in sexual stimulation and foreplay.

3. Range of motion. Loss of range of motion, particularly about the hips, and especially for a woman, can make normal coitus difficult, if not impossible. The physician should particularly check for hip flexion contractures and abduction. The "mechanical barrier" in patients is important, especially with involvement of the hip joints. The Faber Maneuver (an acronym for flexion, abduction, and external rotation of the hips) performed with the patient supine is helpful in identifying mechanical limitations which may interfere with coitus and which often are amenable to surgery. Testing for hip and pelvic mobility presents another appropriate time to initiate questions about sexual activity and satisfaction, or to raise additional questions based on physical findings.

4. Pain. Movements and areas of pain should be identified, as should movements and positions which relieve discomfort.

DIAGNOSIS

In establishing the diagnosis, it is helpful to distinguish between primary and secondary sexual dysfunction.

Primary

Primary dysfunction refers to any long-standing problem which has been present for most of an individual's adolescent and adult life (for example, a male who has never had an erection). Patients with primary dysfunctions should be referred to a specialist.

Secondary

Secondary dysfunction refers to problems that have a fairly recent onset, such as intermittent or situational impotence. Such sexual problems may be either unrelated, related to, or aggravated by the patient's physical disability. Patients with a secondary dysfunction, which comprise the largest group, can often be treated quite successfully by the family practitioner.

PRINCIPLES OF MANAGEMENT

General Approach

P-LI-SS-IT Model. This is a simple but effective strategy for dealing with patients with sexual dysfunctions. It provides an increasing order of complexity and sophistication for involvement, but in general does not depend on specialized training and skill in sexual counseling or therapy. It is designed for patients with secondary sexual dysfunctions. The acronym P-LI-SS-IT stands for " Permission, Limited Information, Specific Suggestions, and Intensive Therapy." Each is described briefly as follows:

1. Permission. Many patients simply require the permission or sanction of an authority figure or someone they respect to become sexually active or to try different options in coping with disability.

2. Limited Information. Frequently, all that patients require is a simple explanation of anatomical or physiologic issues, which gives them adequate knowledge to make informed decisions and allays their fears and anxieties.

3. Specific Suggestions. See the basic guidelines below and the suggestions listed under the individual disorders discussed later in the chapter.

4. Intensive Therapy. Patients who require intensive therapy should generally be referred to a specialist. This will include patients with pri-

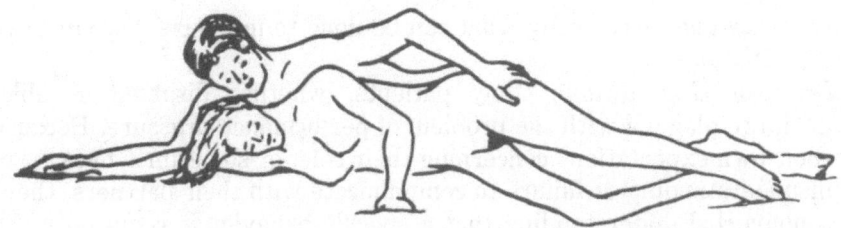

FIG. 4. When spine immobility is a problem, couples may find the side-by-side position easier, either face-to-face or back-to-front as shown (from Anderson et al., 1979).

mary sexual dysfunctions and others who do not respond to the earlier steps in the P-LI-SS-IT Model.

Basic Guidelines

Timing   Identify the time of day and the set of circumstances when pain, spasticity, or other symptoms which interfere with sexual activity are least severe. Suggest that the patient plan sexual activity around these times. The physician should also explore altering the medication schedule so that the period of maximum effectiveness coincides with planned sexual activity. For example, changing the schedule of pain medication for a patient with arthritis can often be very helpful.

Position   Patients need to experiment with a variety of positions to discover which requires the least expenditure of energy and is most comfortable. For many couples, the side-by-side positions (Figure 4) are the most satisfactory (either face-to-face or back-to-front), especially when spine and hip mobility present problems.

Barriers to Mobility   Question the patient to find out what types of things are most effective in reducing spasticity, pain, and other barriers to mobility. If heat is effective, for example, suggest that the patient take a warm bath before sexual activity, preferably with his or her partner. Water beds and massage oils may help to reduce friction and fatigue for the person with severe joint limitations or in whom repeated movement causes discomfort.

Nonsexual Activities   Some of the best clues about what provides effective physical relief and comfort can be obtained by exploring nonsexual activity and discovering what can be done to minimize discomfort in these situations.

Level of Expectation Many patients, whether disabled or able-bodied, are plagued with the problem of performance pressure. Because of their own expectations concerning their role, or sometimes because of a misunderstanding or failure to communicate with their partners, there is a nonverbal understanding that a specific behavior is required when this, in fact, is not the case. Encouraging couples to discuss their expectations of one another candidly and openly, and then giving them assignments which minimize the focus on genital play or achieving orgasm, can be extremely helpful.

Partners Chronic illness places special demands on the nondisabled partner. Open, honest communication becomes especially important. If possible, the physician should talk with the partner alone and then together with the patient. Some questions to ask include: "What is the partner's perception of the dysfunction?" "What are the partner's attitudes about the patient's disability?" "Is the partner as sexually active and satisfied as he or she would like to be?" When the patient is severely impaired, there is often an unrecognized problem for the sexual partner, who also plays a major care provider role. Many patients have found that having a third person be the care provider at certain times relieves the sexual partner of that responsibility, and gives him or her more time and energy to concentrate on the sexual role.

Information It is surprising how many myths patients have about how their bodies function. A special concern of disabled patients is whether certain activities will be harmful. Providing basic information about the disability as well as the anatomy and physiology of sexual function can relieve unnecessary apprehension and fears.

Attitudes For most persons, whether able-bodied or disabled, attitudes present the largest barrier to achieving a satisfactory sexual adjustment. Helping patients reassess their sexual attitudes can be a very effective therapeutic measure.

Drugs Numerous drugs interfere with sexual function. A partial list of these is shown in Table 3.

MANAGEMENT OF SPECIFIC DISORDERS

Heart Disease

General Information The major concerns in advising patients with heart disease about sexual activities are related to energy expenditure

TABLE 3. DRUGS WHICH INTERFERE WITH SEXUAL FUNCTION

Antihypertensives

Diuretics
   spironolactone—decreases testosterone; gynecomastia
   methyldopa—impotence
Others
   guanethidine—decreases erection, ejaculation, vaginal lubrication
   hydralazine—decreases erection, vaginal lubrication
   glycosides—decreases testosterone; gynecomastia

Tranquilizers

Phenothiazines—decreases erection, ejaculation
Benzodiazepines—galactorrhea, impotence (more with chlordiazepoxide than diazepam)

Antidepressants

Tricyclic
   amitriptyline—decreases libido and intensity of orgasms; galactorrhea; testicular, breast
      swelling

Miscellaneous

Mecamylamine—impotence
Phenoxybenzamine—decreases ejaculation
Propantheline—impotence

and oxygen consumption. Until fairly recently, physicians were able to counsel their patients with only vague generalizations and guidelines. However, with the advent of cardiac stress testing and Holter-type monitoring, our understanding of cardiac functioning during the sexual response cycle has expanded enormously. This means that most patients can be provided with specific information and guidelines.

Of the four phases of the sexual response cycle—excitement, plateau, orgasm, and resolution—the maximum stress on the cardiopulmonary system occurs during orgasm. In young, healthy persons, heart rates commonly go as high as 170, and respiratory rates range from 30–60 breaths per minute. By contrast, however, it has been shown that the stress is considerably less in middle-aged men with arteriosclerotic heart disease who are having intercourse with their wives. The mean heart rate during orgasm for one such group of men was 117, with an average of 98 beats per minute, two minutes before and two minutes after orgasm.

The best way to develop a specific prescription for any physical exertion, including sexual activity, is with one of the standard exercise stress tests using either a treadmill or bicycle ergometer. As a general rule, activities should be limited to heart rates which stay below 75–85 percent of the maximum recorded during the stress test. Another common method for prescribing a person's activity level is in terms of mets,* which correlate well with the heart rate; this is a simple method of determining oxygen consumption. While engaged in intercourse, energy expenditure reaches 5 mets for less than 30 seconds during orgasm and is approximately 3.7 mets just prior to and after orgasm. Therefore, a cardiac patient who can walk on a treadmill at three to four miles per hour without symptoms or significant changes in blood pressure or ECG should be able to engage safely in sexual activity. If necessary, a more specific prescription can be developed by employing the Sexercise Tolerance Test. For this test, a Holter Monitor is worn for 24 hours, including a period of usual sexual activity. With the aid of a diary kept by the patient, ECG changes can be correlated with specific activities and levels of exertion.

Specific Suggestions

1. When to resume sexual activity. There is no agreement as to the best time to resume sexual activity. General guidelines recommended by most authorities are from two to six weeks following coronary artery surgery, and six weeks after myocardial infarction.

2. Position. One study has shown that, contrary to popular belief, the male inferior position is not significantly different from the male superior position in terms of energy expenditure. Although the side-to-side position would seem less strenuous, this has not been studied.

3. Partner. The quality of the relationship the patient has with his or her partner is an important consideration in providing appropriate guidance and counsel. It has been shown that clandestine extramarital activities are associated with a high occurrence of myocardial infarctions. At the same time, an unhappy marital relationship can be the source of considerable stress as well. A compatible, understanding, caring partner can help minimize the stress and anxiety of resuming sexual activity. Counseling the patient and partner together is often effective in facilitating their communication and understanding of each other's needs.

4. Fatigue. Patients should engage in sexual activities when well rested. Fatigue impairs sexual function and more cardiac work may be required to achieve satisfaction.

*One met is the energy expenditure per kilogram of body weight per minute of an average individual sitting quietly in a chair or lying at rest. Walking three to four miles per hour is equivalent to five or six mets.

5. Eating. Patients should wait at least three hours after a heavy meal before engaging in sexual activity because of the demands of digestion on the heart.

6. Alcohol. Alcohol intake should be reduced prior to sex. Alcohol increases the peripheral circulation, but reduces coronary circulation. In addition, the CNS depressant effects of alcohol have an inhibitory effect on the libido, often necessitating increased work to accomplish sexual fulfillment.

7. Temperature. The room temperature should be as comfortable as possible. Temperature extremes, especially with high humidity, increase cardiac work.

8. Physical conditioning. Sexual activity is favorably influenced by improving the level of physical fitness. Patients should be encouraged to engage in cardiac conditioning programs whenever possible.

9. Drugs. Many medications taken by patients with heart disease may cause or aggravate sexual problems or dysfunctions. Reducing the dosage or changing the medication schedule may minimize some of the side-effects. Examples of drugs which are commonly associated with sexual dysfunctions are: guanethidine, which may cause retrograde ejaculations; and pentolinium, mecamylamine, and methyldopa, which may delay or inhibit ejaculation.

10. Warning signs. Patients should be advised concerning important warning signs which may occur during sexual activity. These include chest pains during or after sex, palpitations or breathlessness that continue for 15 minutes after coitus, and severe exhaustion that persists into the day following sexual activity.

Stroke

General Information In contrast to heart disease, there is much less information available about the physiologic changes and metabolic demands associated with sexual activity following a stroke. As a result, it is more difficult to provide patients with specific guidelines or suggestions. As a general rule, however, unless cerebral damage is very severe, the sexual response, both anatomically and neurologically, is usually spared. The level of sexual interest and activity in stroke victims has not been extensively studied. However, in one group of 105 stroke patients under 60 years of age, the majority reported having some subjective sexual desire but a decreased opportunity to satisfy that desire. Of the patients in the study, 60 percent had the same or greater sexual interest following the stroke, compared to their level of interest before the onset of disability; 43 percent had a decreased frequency of coitus, while 22 percent had an increased frequency of intercourse.

Specific Suggestions

1. Sensory. Maximize areas of preserved sensation. Since many stroke patients have sensory deficits, both the stroke victim and his or her partner should be encouraged to focus erotic stimulation and love play on those areas of the body with normal sensation. As with any other disability, partners should be encouraged to explore and experiment to discover what provides the most pleasure. Partners also need to be informed if there are any visual deficits, such as homonomous hemianopsia, so they can make appropriate adjustments in their positions or movements.

2. Motor. Use positions of maximum comfort which require a minimum of stress on weakened or impaired muscles. An overhead trapeze, a handle on the headboard, and firm pillows or cushions are simple, effective means to facilitate moving or positioning in bed.

Arthritis

General Information   Satisfactory sexual adjustment in arthritis patients poses the same problems as in persons without a physical handicap. Chronic arthritis, however, presents additional problems, especially in three key areas. First, the nature of a sexual dysfunction is likely to be more difficult to diagnose since it is frequently complicated by the underlying medical condition. Second, successful intervention is more elusive because of the fluctuating physical and emotional factors often associated with arthritis. Third, as with other long-term disabilities, arthritis places special stresses on the patient's sexual partner and on their relationship. Many patients report that it is often easier for them than for their partner to accept limitations or explore alternative forms of sexual expression, because they have had to deal more directly with the problem of coping and adapting with their disability in other areas. Thus, involving the partner is especially critical in assessing and managing sexual dysfunctions in arthritic patients.

Since pain is a predominant problem in all forms of arthritis, most of the suggestions discussed refer to that symptom; however, the principles may apply to other symptoms as well.

Specific Suggestions

1. Preparation. Sexual activities are frequently fatiguing. This can provoke pain and tenderness in joints and muscles, which can then act as a disincentive to further sexual intimacy. Therefore, patients should be advised to do some simple warm-up exercises to prepare their bodies for

the extra exertion anticipated in a sexual encounter. Moist heat is often an effective adjunct which provides additional analgesia and relaxation as part of the preparatory activities.

2. Barriers to mobility. Discover what works best to relieve or reduce pain and then encourage the patient to schedule his or her sexual activities around that relief. For example, if heat is effective, suggest that the patient take a warm bath before engaging in sex, preferably with his or her partner. For patients with severe joint limitations or in whom repetitious movements cause discomfort, water beds and massage oils can help reduce friction and fatigue. In advanced stages of arthritis, total joint replacements may be extremely beneficial in restoring the necessary mobility to permit resumption of satisfactory sexual relations.

3. Timing. Identify the time of day and circumstances when pain or other symptoms which lessen sexual interest and desire are least severe. Suggest that the patient plan his or her sexual activity around these times. You might also consider altering the medication schedule so that the period of maximum effectiveness coincides with planned sexual activity.

4. Position. Suggest that the patient try a variety of positions to discover which is most comfortable and requires the least exertion. Many couples have found that the side-by-side positions (see Figure 4) are the most satisfactory (either face-to-face, or back-to-front), especially when spine and hip mobility are problems.

Neuromuscular disorders

General Information   There are a large number of disorders of the neuromuscular systems which have a lasting and profound effect on sexual function and performance. Some of the more common include multiple sclerosis, amyotrophic lateral sclerosis, muscular dystrophy, spina bifida, cerebral palsy, and spinal cord injury. Although each of these has its own characteristic set of problems and complications, the purpose of this section is to deal with some of the sexual issues which are common to these and other neuromuscular disorders. With the exception of multiple sclerosis and spinal cord injuries, there is relatively little information available on physical and neurological changes that affect sexual functioning in these disorders; most of the data that do exist are based on studies of men.

A case in point is a study of 37 men with multiple sclerosis, which correlates pseudomotor activity and potency. Patients who were totally impotent sweated normally to the waist, but not below; subjects who were partially impotent sweated normally to the groin and perineum, but not in the lower extremities. By contrast, patients with good potency exhibited normal sweating throughout the body. It was also noted that changes in both potency and sweating correlated with clinical remissions and relapses.

Sexual functioning has been studied fairly extensively in men with spinal cord injuries. Table 4 summarizes a number of reports with regard to reflex erections, anteriograde ejaculation, coital success, and fertility. Patients with incomplete lesions (sparing of motor and/or sensory function below the level of injury) are more likely to have preserved function in these areas than are patients with complete lesions, regardless of whether they are upper motor neuron or lower motor neuron lesions. Reflex erections are more common in patients with upper motor neuron lesions, regardless of completeness; that is, in lesions which are more likely to spare the reflex arc which is mediated by the sacral cord (S2-4). Ejaculation, which is mediated by sympathetic and somatic fibers, occurs most commonly in patients with incomplete lower motor neuron injuries, while coital success generally parallels the figures reported for reflex erections. In this group of men, the percentage who fathered offspring ranged from one to ten percent. As indicated in Table 2, information regarding the sexual response in women with spinal cord injuries is incomplete. In terms of fertility, however, it is important to counsel patients that the spinal injury does not alter ability to conceive; these patients have the same physiologic potential for becoming pregnant as they had prior to injury. For this reason, female patients who are contemplating becoming sexually active should take appropriate precautions to avoid unwanted pregnancies.

Specific Suggestions

1. Preparation. Cleanliness is especially important for persons who wear catheters, leg bags, or other devices. Persons who do not have normal or voluntary control of bowel and bladder should generally plan a bowel and bladder evacuation prior to sexual activity so that the possibility of an accident is minimized.

2. Indwelling catheters. Catheters do not always have to be removed for either males or females. In the male, the catheter can be bent and folded along the shaft of the penis and either covered with a condom or left uncovered. Either way, the penis and catheter can be readily inserted into the vagina and, if well lubricated, should not be a source of irritation. For the female, the catheter can be positioned to one side and need not interfere with foreplay or penile-vaginal intercourse.

3. External catheter. These are usually removed prior to sexual activ-

TABLE 4. SEXUAL FUNCTION IN MEN WITH SPINAL CORD LESIONS*

Lesion	Psychogenic Erection	Reflex Erection	Anteriograde Ejaculation	Coital Success	Orgasm	Progeny
UMN, Complete	0	90–95	<7	70	rare	1–3
UMN, Incomplete	25	95–100	30	80–85	occasional	5–10
LMN, Complete	25	25	20	70	occasional-common	5–10
LMN, Incomplete	80–85	90	70	90	common	10

UMN = upper motor neuron
LMN = lower motor neuron

*figures represent percent occurrence

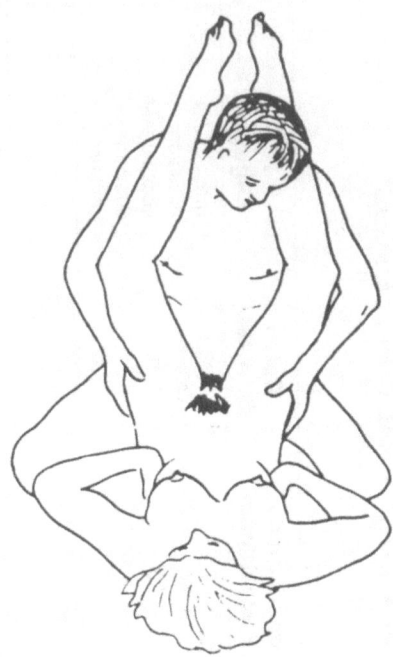

FIG. 5. This position might be used if the range of motion at the hips and/or knees is limited (from Anderson et al., 1979).

ity. However, as mentioned earlier, prior to removal of the catheter or just prior to initiating foreplay, the bladder should be emptied using a Credé maneuver or other technique.

4. Assistance. For some patients, the lack of strength and physical dexterity often requires the assistance of another person in achieving a certain position or in putting on or taking off various devices like condoms or catheters. Many patients have found that having a third person— usually a trained attendant—assist with some of these procedures is helpful in facilitating preparation, and relieves the able-bodied partner of some of the "nursing role." This obviously requires a lot of candid discussion on the part of all concerned.

5. Foreplay. Partners should create an environment conducive to sexual stimulation and enjoyment. Key points include privacy, lighting (perhaps with candles), special smells (for example, incense), sound (relaxing,

romantic music), and tastes (food, drink). The physician should encourage patients to discover what is pleasurable and to experiment.

6. Impotence. As mentioned previously, patients with lesions at the sacral cord have the least chance of reflex erections, while those with lesions in the thoracic and cervical cord have the greatest possibility of erections. Patients in whom this reflex is intact may find that they can facilitate and prolong erections by stimulating the scrotum or by mildly irritating the testicular sac, inner thigh, pubic hair, or anal area. An erection that is not completely full or hard can still be inserted into the vagina using the "stuffing" technique. In this technique, the disabled man assumes the dominant position, and with his fingers and the help of his partner, stuffs the flaccid, soft penis into the vaginal opening. This sometimes will produce a reflex erection, especially if the woman is able to thrust her hips forward and squeeze the vaginal muscles around the penis.

7. Accessories. A water bed may be helpful, especially with high-level disability, because the motion of the mattress can facilitate movement during foreplay and intercourse. If finger and hand strength and dexterity are impaired, a vibrator can be strapped to the forearm and used to pleasure the partner.

8. Lubrication. Many women with spinal injuries report a decreased

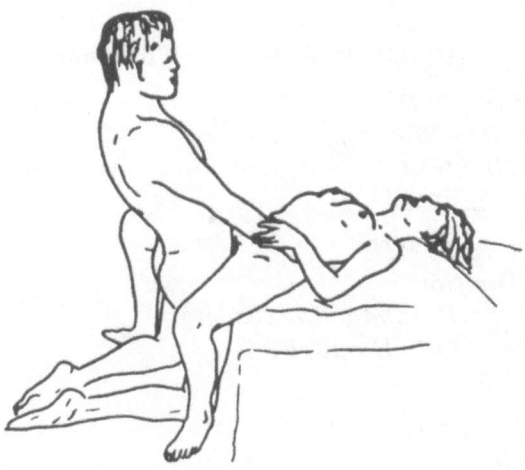

FIG. 6. This position is an alternative for the person with reduced strength, endurance, or coordination (from Anderson et al., 1979).

lubrication of the vagina. This can be supplemented with the use of a lubrication material like K-Y Jelly.

9. Contraception. For patients with impaired mobility, there is usually an increased risk of thrombophlebitis. For this reason, oral contraceptives are generally not the contraceptive of choice; however, the risks and benefits of this type of contraceptive should be weighed against those of other contraceptive techniques. For women with impaired function of the fingers and hands, insertion of a diaphragm may be impractical. Likewise, patients with impaired sensation in the genital and pelvic area usually are not good candidates for IUDs. In these patients, a condom worn by the man may be the most practical and sensible approach to contraception.

10. Contractures. (See "Barriers to Mobility" under "Arthritis.") For a woman with contractures at the hips and knees, the position shown in Figure 5 can be tried, with her hips over her partner's shoulders.

11. Decreased strength and endurance. If the able-bodied partner is a woman, one possibility is to use the female-astride position. If the woman is disabled and has an able-bodied male partner, one suggestion is to have her lie supine with him kneeling on the bed or floor, as shown in Figure 6.

APPENDIX

A. *List of Sexual Attitude Reassessment Workshops*

Joan Bardach, PhD
Institute of Rehabilitation Medicine
400 East 34th Street
New York, NY 10016

Joseph T. Capell, MD
Assistant Director
Leon S. Peters Rehabilitation Center
Fresno Community Hospital
Fresno, CA 93702

Theodore Cole, MD
Sandra Cole
Department of Physical Medicine and Rehabilitation
University of Michigan
School of Medicine
Ann Arbor, MI 48109

Stanley Ducharme, PhD
Boston University School of Medicine
75 East Newton Street
New England Spinal Cord Injury Center
Boston, MA 02118

Benita Fifield
Department of Occupational Therapies
Faculty of Rehabilitation Medicine
University of Alberta
Edmonton, Alberta, Canada T6G2G4

Orville Fifield
Alberta Institute of Human Sexuality
244 Westridge Road
Edmonton, Alberta, Canada T5T1C1

Dorothea Glass, MD
Medical Director
Moss Rehabilitation Hospital
12th and Tabor Road
Philadelphia, PA 19141

Winona Griggs
Rehabilitation Institute of Chicago
345 East Superior—16th Floor
Chicago, IL 60611

Lauro Halstead, MD
Kris Halstead, MS
The Institute for Rehabilitation and Research
1333 Moursund Avenue
Houston, TX 77030

Scott Manley, EdD
Cathy Manley
Craig Hospital
Family Service Department
3425 South Clarkson
Englewood, CO 80110

Dan Mayclin, PhD
Santa Clara Valley Medical Center
751 South Bascom Avenue
San Jose, CA 95128

B. *Sources for Information, Films, Books, and Pamphlets*
   on Sexuality and Disability

   American Association of Sex Educators, Counselors and Therapists
   (AASECT)
   5010 Wisconsin Avenue, NW, Suite 304
   Washington, DC 20016

   Multi Media Resource Center
   1525 Franklin Street
   San Francisco, CA 94109
   (films, videotapes)

   Planned Parenthood Federation of America
   Alan Guttmacher Institute
   515 Madison Avenue
   New York, NY 10022

   Sex Information and Education Council of the United States
   (SIECUS)
   1855 Broadway
   New York, NY 10028

REFERENCES

Anderson F, Bardach J, Goodgold J: *Sexuality and Neuromuscular Disease.* Rehabilitation Monograph No. 56. New York, Institute of Rehabilitation Medicine, and Muscular Dystrophy Association, 1979

Cole TM: Sexuality and the Spinal Cord Injured. In: Green, R (ed) Human Sexuality. A Health Practitioner's Text. Baltimore. Williams and Wilkins, 1975

Comfort, A: *Sexual Consequences of Disability.* Philadelphia, George F. Stickley Co, 1978

Halstead, LS, Halstead, MG, Salhoot, JT, et al: Sexual attitudes, behavior and satisfaction for able-bodied and disabled participants attending workshops in sexuality. *Arch Phys Med Rehab* 59: 497–501, 1978

Hellerstein, H, Friedman, EH: Sexual activity and the postcoronary patient. *Med Asp Hum Sex,* 3(3):70–96, 1969.

Masters WH, Johnson VE: *Human Sexual Response.* Boston, Little, Brown & Co, 1966

Mooney, TO, Cole TM, Chilgren RA: *Sexual Options for Paraplegics and Quadriplegics.* Boston, Little, Brown & Co, 1975

Sadoughi, S, et al: Sexual adjustment in a chronically ill and physically disabled population: A pilot study. *Arch Phy Med Rehab* 52: 311, 1971

8

The Problem of Pornography

Morris A. Lipton

The mere appearance of the topic of pornography in a volume devoted to the phenomenology and treatment of psychosexual disorders immediately reflects several existing conflicting views about the existence of a pornographic industry in our society. One view is that exposure to pornography leads to immorality. To politically conservative and religious groups, this immorality is associated with loss of interest in traditional values, such as belief in God, patriotism, and the sanctity of the family. Associated with such decline in morality, they claim there is increasing promiscuity, illegitimacy, abortion rates, drug use, and both nonsexual and sexual crime.

A variant of this conservative position is held by some otherwise liberal feminist groups who feel that exposure to pornography is degrading. They say it debases and dehumanizes women, making them objects of male dominance rather than human beings. A consequence of this, they state, is that there is an increase in exploitation and violent sexual crimes against women. Some feminists distinguish between erotica and pornography and wish to permit the former while banning the latter. Both contain explicit sex but the former exists in an equal loving context, the latter in a demeaning or violent context. Other feminists see all explicit sex portrayed by women in magazines and movies as de facto degrading and hence pornographic (Steinem, 1980; Brownmiller, 1975).

A second view held by many liberals is that pornography is a relatively mild psychosexual stimulant which offers entertainment to some individuals, does no harm, and often may release sexual tension for the

113

lonely. These liberals believe it may even have some educational and therapeutic value for the sexually inhibited.

Proponents of the first view generally tend to favor strict federal and state laws prohibiting the production, distribution, and sales of pornography. Proponents of the latter view want no federal laws and wish to minimize even local statutes; they prefer to permit individuals and communities which see pornography as a nuisance or evil to use extra-legal methods like sex education or community boycotts and other social pressures to control it.

Underlying the conflicts between conservative moralists and liberals, there has always been the problem of the First Amendment—the right to freedom of expression. Liberals believe that a fundamental right in a democratic society is the right to free speech. This right must be carefully protected to permit the expression of divergent and unpopular views. It is limited, all liberals would agree, only by the question of whether the material uttered, written, or displayed creates a "clear and present danger." Thus, as Justice Oliver Wendell Holmes once said, it does not permit the right to yell "fire" in a crowded theatre. The liberals are greatly concerned that if this right is tampered with at all, censorship will take over and books will be banned or burned. There is some legitimacy in this concern because at various times authors like Chaucer, Boccaccio, Dostoyevsky, Mark Twain, James Joyce, Thomas Mann, J. D. Salinger, and Kurt Vonnegut have been on right wing "hit lists" with demands that they be removed from public and school libraries. To such moralists, some of the works of these authors represent a "clear and present danger" to our national traditions and religious values and are, therefore, not fully protected by the First Amendment. Some would expurgate this literature, others would limit the circulation to adults.

The problem of what to do about pornography is not new. In the English speaking world, it goes back about 300 years. Legal restrictions with punishment have been tried repeatedly with little long-term success. The importance of the problem and the intensity of the demand for solutions waxes and wanes at apparently unpredictable intervals. The typical moralist solution is to create religious sanctions and secular laws and enforce them rigorously; the liberal solution is to tolerate pornography and its users under First Amendment protection and to permit it unless there is evidence that it enhances criminal sexual behavior. In 1967, the US Congress felt the problem to be of sufficient magnitude to appropriate funds and to petition President Lyndon Johnson to establish a commission whose function was, "after a thorough study which shall include a study of the causal relationship of such material to antisocial behavior, to recommend advisable, appropriate, and constitutional means to deal effectively with such traffic in obscenity and pornography."

THE COMMISSION ON OBSCENITY AND PORNOGRAPHY

Composition, Strategies & Conclusions

In 1968, the Commission on Obscenity and Pornography was established. Of its 18 members appointed by President Johnson, five were attorneys or judges; four were concerned with the publication and dissemination of books, movies, and television programs; three were clergymen of the Protestant, Catholic, and Jewish faiths; three were sociologists; two were psychiatrists; and one was an educator. One commissioner resigned to become Ambassador to India; his replacement was the only appointment made by President Richard Nixon.

The strategy of the Commission followed the specific tasks assigned to it by the Congress in Public Law 90-100. Four separate panels with specific duties were established. The task of the legal panel was "to analyze the laws pertaining to the control of obscenity and pornography, and to recommend definitions of obscenity and pornography." A traffic and distribution panel attempted to "ascertain the methods employed in the distribution of obscene and pornographic material and to explore the nature and volume of traffic in such material." The role of the effects panel was "to study the effect of obscenity and pornography upon the public and particularly minors, and its relationship to crime and other antisocial behavior." The effects panel limited itself to the question of the influence of exposure to erotic material on sexual attitudes, conduct, and mental health. It did not attempt to measure effects (if any) on political or religious persuasion.

A positive approach panel undertook to "recommend such legislative, administrative or other advisable and appropriate action as the Commission deems necessary to regulate effectively the flow of such traffic, without in any way interfering with constitutional rights."

The work of the Commission generated more information about the nature of the industry, the characteristics of users, and the consequences of exposure than previously had been available in this nation. The findings, conclusions, and recommendations, entitled *The Report of The Commission on Obscenity and Pornography*, were published in 1970. The report was supplemented with nine published volumes of technical documents which contained the data on which the report was based. Since both conservatives and liberals buttress their ideological stances with claims of demonstrable damaging or innocuous effects of pornography, the full commission depended greatly on the data generated by the effects panel in determining its recommendation. If detrimental effects of pornography could be documented, the position of moralists would have been strengthened and the panel presumably would have recommended restrictive legislation. Based on the data available at that time, the effects panel was unable to find persuasive evidence that pornography presented a "clear and present danger." In their report, the effects panel wrote . . . "if a case is to be made against 'pornography' in 1970, it will have to be made on grounds other than effects of a damaging personal or social nature."

The Commission struggled with a definition of pornography, as others had before, but was unable to establish a rigorous one. Instead, it used a guideline of "verbal or pictorial representations of sexual behavior that have as a distinguishing characteristic the degrading and demeaning portrayal of the role and status of the human female . . . as a mere sexual object to be exploited and manipulated sexually." These guidelines were not without their problems. A degrading and demeaning portrayal, like pornography itself, is often in the eye and mind of the beholder. To some, the fact that an actress would perform sexually before a camera is de facto evidence of such behavior no matter what the context (Brownmiller, 1975).

The Commission, on the basis of the evidence collected, concluded that the possibly demeaning content of pornography did not adversely affect male actions toward women. The position of the majority of the Commission was that, while pornography may be vulgar and tasteless, it basically is an entertainment that harms no one but its consumers, who may at worst suffer from the debasement of their tastes. Legislation controlling pornography would be an unjustifiable abridgement of the rights of freedom of speech of those who make and distribute pornographic materials and of the rights of privacy of their customers. The Commission, by a vote of 12 to 6, opined that "federal, state, and local legislation prohibiting the sale, exhibition, and distribution of sexual materials to consenting adults should be repealed." The Report of the Commission and its recommendations have been acclaimed in the liberal community and by many clinicians, juvenile workers, and behavioral scientists.

The minority position—to retain existing legislation at all levels and to enforce the laws more vigorously—was supported by the three clergymen, the attorney general of California, the Nixon appointee who was the director of a national antipornography organization, and a woman educator. Several of those favored stronger legislation, especially at the federal level. Vice President Spiro Agnew said that neither he nor President Nixon would permit "Main Street to be converted to Smut Alley." President Nixon stated that "I have evaluated the report and categorically reject its morally bankrupt conclusions." Many popular religious leaders and conservative politicians and journalists agreed.

The Commission also made several other legal and nonlegal recommendations which are often forgotten. They are listed below.

Recommendations of the Majority of the Commission

A. *Legal*

1. It recommended that federal, state, and local legislation prohibiting the sale, exhibition, or distribution of sexual materials for consenting adults should be repealed.

2. It recommended and prepared model state statutes prohibiting the commercial distribution or display for sale of sexual materials to young persons.

3. It recommended enactment of state and local legislation prohibiting public display of sexually explicit pictorial materials and approved the existing federal legislation regarding the mailing of unsolicited advertisements of a sexually explicit nature.

4. It recommended legislation authorizing prosecutors to obtain declaratory judgments as to whether particular materials fall within existing legal prohibitions and appropriate injunctive relief. This would make prosecution primarily civil except where the materials at issue are unquestionably within the applicable statutory definitional provisions.

5. It recommended against any legislation which would limit or abolish the jurisdiction of the Supreme Court or other federal courts in obscenity cases.

B. *Nonlegal*

1. That a massive sex education program be launched.

2. That there be continued open discussion, based on factual information on the issues regarding obscenity and pornography.

3. That additional factual information be obtained through continued research.

4. That citizens organize themselves at local, regional, and national levels to aid in the implementation of the foregoing recommendations.

Evidence on Effects-1970

The effects panel used multiple approaches simultaneously to address the question of whether the distribution of explicit sexually arousing material might constitute a "clear and present danger" causing delinquent or criminal sexual behavior among youth and adults. Details of its methods and findings are available in the Commission Report (1970) and in Volume VII of its Technical Reports. A brief summary by this author is available elsewhere (Lipton, 1976), and an even briefer summary is presented here.

1. The existing research literature on the effects of sexually arousing material on behavior was very sparse in 1970. Research prior to the formation of the Commission was limited to immediate sexual arousal responses and failed to consider how this arousal might affect behavior. It showed that a large proportion of adults could become sexually aroused by pictures and words. The Commission research showed that arousing sexual stimuli for women differed from that of men, ie, stories were generally more arousing than pictures. The social context of the viewing significantly determined the extent of arousal.

2. The effects panel examined the popular literature and the writing of "experts" and found a wide range of opinions, none of which were supported by satisfactory data. Some experts felt that exposure is harmful to people; some felt that it was harmless or beneficial. In general, law enforcement officials tended to see pornography as more dangerous than did behavioral scientists, but a few well-known psychiatrists had strong opinions that erotica had damaging effects.

3. The Commission sponsored a questionnaire which was submitted to 3500 psychiatrists and clinical psychologists on the question of whether, in their experience, exposure to pornography was related to antisocial sexual behavior. Eighty percent reported that they had never encountered such a case, nine percent suspected such cases, and seven percent were convinced that there was a relationship. When asked whether reading obscene books plays a significant role in causing juvenile delinquency, professional workers, child guidance counselors, and social workers in psychology responded with 77 percent "no," 10 percent "don't know," and 12 percent "yes." In contrast, police chiefs responded to the same questions with 31 percent "no," 11 percent "don't know," and 58 percent "yes."

4. A public opinion survey involving 2500 adults and 769 persons in the 15–20-year-old age range asked the question, "Will you please tell me

what you think are the two or three most serious problems facing the country today?" Only two percent answered concern about erotic materials. The majority was much more concerned with the Vietnam War, state of the economy, racial conflict, or drug abuse. The same survey revealed that a large majority of the adults and youth surveyed had had experience with specifically erotic materials. When asked whether they wished greater legal controls on pornography that would limit availability, about one third of the public favored such controls even if no harm could be demonstrated, while more than 50 percent opposed greater restriction unless it could be shown that the material was harmful. These results contrast with those from a Gallup and Harris Poll in 1969 that revealed that 75–85 percent of adults wanted stricter laws on pornography. In response to a series of questions as to what erotica did to people, a wide divergence of opinions was elicited. In general, positive or neutral effects of explicit sexual materials were associated with higher levels of education, greater exposure, and relative youth. Older, less educated, and sexually conservative people tended to see more undesirable effects. Most respondents judged that such materials had more benign or neutral effects on themselves but possibly more damaging effects on others.

5. Direct experiments were conducted to determine the nature of arousing materials. These experiments showed that from 60–85 percent of both men and women experienced sexual arousal when reading or viewing certain erotic stimuli. Women were more aroused by written material and less stimulated by visual material. Most sexual scenes of petting and heterosexual coitus were equally arousing to both sexes but group oral sex was more arousing to men. Incarcerated sexual offenders tended to be aroused by the same types of materials as control subjects, but sexual deviants responded to literary or depicted stimuli similar to those that they encountered in real life. Thus, transvestite men were likely to find clothing more erotic than nudity or coitus. For pedophils, the popular advertisement for a tanning lotion showing a dog tugging at the panties of a child was more arousing than a *Playboy* centerfold. Arousal during exposure diminishes with age.

6. A direct experiment on male college students showed that repeated heavy exposure to erotica rapidly leads to satiation and boredom. Such exposure did not significantly affect sleep, mood, study, or work habits. It did not alter the nature or amount of the subject's personal sexual activities. Such heavy exposure led to increases in sexual dreams and sexual conversation for a brief time.

7. Retrospective examinations of sex offenders were conducted. Delin-

quent and nondelinquent youths tended to have the same time, nature, and extent of exposure to erotica. Both groups had considerable experience with such materials. Adult sex offenders respond to erotic materials to about the same degree as does a control population; however, the comparison of incarcerated sex offenders and nonsex offenders reveals that rapists had their first exposure to erotica at age 18 and nonsex offenders at age 15. In general, sex offenders report sexually repressive background and immature and inadequate sexual histories as well as less and later exposure to erotica than control subjects.

8. The Danish experience following liberalization of their laws on distribution of pornography was evaluated; this indicated somewhat of a decrease and certainly no increase in sex crimes following the repeal of previously existing laws.

Limitations of the Evidence

It should be recognized that the Commission operated under a two-year time constraint in generating the data for its report. It admitted some limitations at the time of publication and retrospectively some other flaws became apparent. For example, the questionnaire in which so few people indicated that concern about pornography was among the two or three most significant issues of the day probably should have asked the respondents to rank order a list, including pornography, of 20 significant issues of the day.* The same poll which showed that most people were tolerant about the question of laws regulating the availability of pornography might have responded differently had they been asked about violent pornography. The satiation experiment was done only on young college men. It would have been better to have replicated the experiment with women and to have extended it to a much wider age range and to different socioeconomic groups. Nonetheless, the results of all of the different types of experiments put together made it clear that there was no evidence to support the proposition that exposure to erotic materials was a significant determining factor in causing sex crimes or delinquency. This was a statistical conclusion, for it was also evident that it would never be possible to state that on no occasion and under no conditions would erotic materials ever contribute in any way to the likelihood of any persons committing a sex crime. The decision to pass prohibitory laws is never

---

*This was done recently with 50 undergraduates of both sexes who attended an evening seminar on this subject. None ranked it among the first 10 issues and only 12 among the top 20. This small number and selected sample makes the results little more than impressionistic data.

based on rare individual cases, but rather on statistical likelihood. On that basis it was not possible to conclude that erotic material is a statistically significant cause of sex crimes. It was on the basis of these findings that the effects panel wrote, "if a case is to be made against pornography in 1970, it will have to be made on grounds other than their effects of a damaging personal nature."

The Commission's recommendation that existing regulations for consenting adults be repealed was based on the absence of detrimental findings plus the survey findings that only about one third of the population was opposed to the distribution of pornography regardless of its effects. On the other hand, it recommended laws against distribution to children, not because children had been tested and shown to be susceptible (for many reasons no such experiments were done), but rather because the public opinion poll showed that a large majority wanted such regulation. By the same reasoning it was felt that people had a right to be protected from material they considered immoral or offensive. Hence, statutes controlling advertising and public display were also recommended. The Commission's recommendation that further research was needed was in large measure due to its awareness of the limitations of the evidence it had generated.

CHANGES IN THE PAST DECADE

Despite the strong recommendation of the Commission for continued research, nothing comparable to its comprehensive effort has been conducted. Thus, there are no systematic surveys about current public attitudes about pornography. It seems fair to say that public concern about it as a highly significant social issue is still low. Although the Vietnam War is no longer a problem, concerns about recession, inflation, and unemployment are now very prominent. The energy crisis, pollution, stability in the Middle East, and international tensions that might lead to a nuclear war would probably be very high on everyone's list. Women have special concerns about equal pay, job discrimination, and their rights to abortion. Effort to pass an Equal Rights Amendment has been a prominent and controversial issue. On the other hand, growth of political conservatism, the emergence of political-religious groups such as the Moral Majority, the continued escalation of violent crime, and the emergence of women's liberation groups that oppose pornography on the grounds that, at the very least, it demeans women, may have raised public concern about pornography to a higher level than it appeared to be in 1970. There are no reliable data on this point. Nor is there evidence that professional opinions about pornography as a cause of sexual crime have altered. Considering the rarity with which even professionals change their positions on issues that have moral content, it appears unlikely.

What is claimed to have changed most is failure of the legal system to protect against pornography, the growth of the pornography industry, the altered content of pornographic materials which increasingly fuse pornography and violence, and the evidence that this mixture does generate reactions and antisocial behavior. These matters will therefore be examined in some detail.

THE LEGAL STATUS OF PORNOGRAPHY

Pornography has ancient origins with vestiges found in Indian, Greek, and Roman art and literature. In the English-speaking world, the ribald stories of Chaucer date back to the fourteenth century. Shakespeare and many other Elizabethan poets used ribaldry frequently. Renaissance art frequently showed erotic paintings and sculpture. The use of obscene language and pornographic themes was common until the 17th century, when during the Puritan influence profanity was prohibited and playhouses were closed. The Puritan influence in the United States resulted in the passage of a statute in 1711 entitled "An Act Against Intemperance, Immorality, and Profaneness in the Reformation of Manners." Note that drinking and profanity were linked, not for medical reasons, but rather for moral and religious ones. For the next two centuries in England and the United States, concern with pornography was never a medical issue but rather a moral one. Medicine entered in only insofar as it was believed that pornography led to depravity and mental illness was a product of such moral depravity. Laws proliferated in England after the Reformation and the rise of Puritanism. The first law to authorize prosecution of obscene materials was enacted in England in 1824. The first conviction dealt with the publishers of a book entitled "Venus in the Cloister or the Nun in her Smock." In the US, blasphemy and other offenses against religion were heavily punished during the 17th and 18th centuries but there are no recorded convictions for the exhibition or sale of purely sexual material until the Fanny Hill case in 1821. Shortly thereafter, Vermont, Connecticut, and Pennsylvania passed anti-obscenity statutes and Massachusetts hardened its laws to define obscene works as "manifestly tending to the corruption of youth." The first federal statute was a customs law of 1842 prohibiting the import of indecent and obscene prints, paintings, and books. In 1865, Congress passed the first law prohibiting the mailing of such material and in 1873 broadened this law to what eventually became its present form. Anthony Comstock was made a special Federal Agent to enforce these laws. By the beginnings of the 20th century, more than 30 states had anti-obscenity legislation.

In 1868, the English courts offered a test to determine whether or not something was pornographic: whether such material "will deprave and corrupt those whose minds are open to such immoral influences." In the United States this test was employed until 1957. During this 100-year period many changes in our society occurred. Dissemination of printed and photographic material increased enormously, and material with sexual content increased correspondingly. Fashions changed to the degree that today's newspaper or magazine ad for underwear or bathing suits would have been considered obscene as recently as 1930, and many of our best selling novels would have been banned. Nudes in magazines became more explicit and "adult" bookstores with books, magazines and "stag" movies proliferated.

Demands for federal control increased so that in 1957 the Supreme Court in the Roth case ruled that "obscenity is not protected within the area of constitutionally protected speech or press." It is worth noting that this decision was not based on the test of "clear and present danger," but rather on the court's judgment that when the Constitution was drafted, states already had statutes prohibiting libel, blasphemy, and profanity, hence the founding fathers could not have meant to constitutionally protect material which was already prohibited in these states. Furthermore, by 1957 all 48 states and 50 other nations had some obscenity laws; from 1842 to 1956, Congress had enacted 20 anti-obscenity laws. To the Court, evidence existed implying a national wish to restrain obscenity.

The Roth decision led to the evolution of a working definition of obscenity. There were three criteria: (1) for the average person, the dominant theme taken as a whole must appeal to a prurient interest in sex; (2) the material must be patently offensive to "contemporary community standards"; and (3) the material must be "utterly" without redeeming social value. This is a marvelously ambiguous set of criteria which points up the difficulties in a strict definition. What is a "community"—a neighborhood, town, county, city, or state? This is a key question for the book publishing and motion picture industries which must operate on estimates of national interest and an anticipated national market. May a book published in New York and distributed throughout the nation be subject to court action in an Iowa community? Could a bookseller or movie house operator be within legal boundaries in Northern California, but trespassing into illegality in Southern California?

What is social value? Entertainment, for example? As expected, the Roth decision led to much litigation and was further confounded by the 1969 decision on Kramer vs Georgia when it was decided that the First and Fourteenth Amendments prohibited making possession of obscene materials a crime. Thus, a person is permitted to legally possess something he may not legally purchase. Finally, in 1973, in the case of Kaplan vs California, the Court by a 5 to 4 decision rejected the recommendation of the 1970 Commission on Obscenity and Pornography that all federal statutes regarding the control of obscene material be lifted. It upheld the Roth decision but changed the definition of obscenity somewhat. The word "utterly" was removed and "serious literacy, artistic, political, or scientific value" was substituted. The Court clearly defined the state as a community, but did not define the smaller limits of a community. The Court also demanded that the nature of the prurient material be described. Only "works which depict or describe sexual conduct" can be outlawed, and that conduct "must be specified by state law." Few states have such specific statutes. Since 1973, more restrictive federal legislation has not been passed.

The problem has obviously not disappeared in the past decade. It is surfacing again partly because of the conservative bend of the country's political climate and partly because of the opposition of new women's rights groups. Both factors point toward a desire for more restrictive legislation.

Since 1970 the results of legal attempts to control pornography have had limited success. Unsolicited advertising through the mail seems to have stopped. Public display of erotic advertisements on billboards, movie theaters, and bookstores seems to have disappeared. Exhibition or sale of pornographic materials to minors seems to be strictly enforced by the merchants who deal with such material. All of these were recommended by the Commission.

The federal laws remain ambiguous. State laws have resulted in a few major convictions like that of Larry Flynt, publisher of *Hustler* magazine. Some movie theaters and some bookstores have been closed, but closings result in lengthy and expensive litigation with few convictions. Most would agree that legal control of pornography for adults has not been effective. Extra-legal community pressure has been more telling in cleaning up neighborhoods. X-rated movies, for example, are usually shown only in drive-in theaters or in sleazy tourist areas, not in residential neighborhoods. "Snuff" films which include rape and murder with disembowelment and dismemberment have had very limited exhibition because of the effectiveness of women's protests (Gever and Hall, 1980; LaBelle, 1980).

The large problem of material for the consenting adult remains. Those who wish stronger legal controls in 1981 make several claims: (1) that the pornography industry has grown enormously, (2) that the content has changed and now contains much violence, (3) that violent pornography is demonstrably dangerous, and (4) that the Pornography Commission was naive, biased, and even dishonest in presenting this evidence. Each of these claims will be examined.

THE SIZE OF THE PORNOGRAPHY INDUSTRY

The traffic panel of the Commission on Pornography studied this problem thoroughly in 1968–1969. It obtained production costs for books, magazines, and movies. It roughly counted the number of bookstores and movie theaters that distributed this material and obtained data about their sales and box office receipts.

This panel concluded that there was no evidence that it was big business. Nudity and erotica that some might call "soft core" pornography, such as that represented in *Playboy, Penthouse,* and R-rated movies, was clearly flourishing, but such materials did not meet the Supreme Court guidelines for prosecution and were, therefore, not the concern of the Commission. "Hard core" pornography was a minor, almost cottage industry type of enterprise. No evidence could be obtained that either organized crime or the major motion picture companies and publishers were involved. Instead, minor entrepreneurs who were able to invest less than $10,000 for the preparation of an erotic book or some tens of thousands of dollars for an X-rated movie, produced and distributed such material in the hope of making a "fast buck." Occasionally they succeeded, as in the cases of "The Devil in Miss Jones" or "Deep Throat," which are still steadily on display in adult movie theatres almost ten years later; however, such successes appear to be very rare.

The traffic panel estimated that in 1970 the pornography industry had total sales of approximately $100 million in the form of adult books, periodicals, mail order items, and under-the-counter material, plus an additional $450 million in the form of box office receipts from both X- and R-rated movies. *Playboy* and similar magazines that are readily available were, in these calculations, not considered pornographic. X-rated films amounted to about seven percent of box office receipts, and unrated sex oriented films about six percent. Since the motion picture industry rates its films to insure compliance with existing federal and state laws so that they may be profitably exhibited in all locales, R-rated films can hardly be classified as hard core pornography. A generous estimate of the hard core pornography industry in 1970 was between $200-350 million.

Claims have been made that in 1980 pornography was a $4 billion per year business (Barry, 1980) protected and controlled in part by organized crime. If this is the case it would represent more than a tenfold increase in ten years and would be sufficiently large to warrant reconsideration of existing statutes and other means of regulation. But no data base similar to that employed by the Commission exists to support these claims.

New systematic research should be conducted in this area, but until then the author must remain skeptical. If the readily available soft core pornography magazines, the many bestseller books which have explicit sexual material, and the multitude of R-rated films are all included it would probably reach or even exceed the $4 billion mark. But, if the definition is limited to those materials available only in adult bookstores and X-rated movies, it is a good guess that the industry remains quite small. These bookstores and movies have not changed much in appearance nor in the volume of business they do. They keep long hours, the run-down movie houses are occupied to not more than ten percent of their capacities, and the bookstores have few browsers and fewer buyers. Related advertisements occupy very little space in newspapers and unsolicited advertising by mail seems to have practically disappeared.

Another estimate is that the pornography industry amounts to $2.5 billion per year with about $1 billion coming from child pornography (Rush, 1980). This estimate is apparently taken from a newspaper feature article titled "Children—A Big Profit Item for Smut Producers." It implies that 25-40 percent of all pornography involves the use of children. This same author estimates that 1.2–1.5 million children under sixteen are involved annually in commercial sex—pornography or prostitution.

In 1970 the Commission encountered very little child pornography and what little there was consisted of still photography imported from poverty stricken countries like India and third world nations. The data base from which these new estimates are made is not offered and it seems incredible that the estimates are correct. It would be very difficult to hide a billion dollar industry involving more than a million children. Moreover, it seems unlikely that there would be so large a market for this type of material. However, if the industry exists even at a level which is only a small portion of these estimates, it is disgraceful. The exploitation of children for prostitution and pornography is not defensible and can and should be prosecuted vigorously under existing laws. To totally wipe it out would probably be impossible because a very small number of children could still be exploited and the capacity to reproduce pictures and films is virtually unlimited. However, existing laws, strictly enforced, would control it greatly.

In summary, unless conclusive contrary data are offered it seems likely to this writer that the pornography industry continues as it has in the past—a marginal industry, too small and too diffuse to warrant the interest of organized crime. Inflation may have generated some total increase in revenue, but this is countered by the recession that might be expected to diminish sales to the usual middle class male consumer. There are rumors that the new video cassette technology which permits permanent possession and viewing in the privacy of one's home may give the pornography business a boost, but no data are available. In short, because of the absence of accurate data at this time, the volume of pornography, the size of the industry, and the nature of the consumer seem to this Ex-Commissioner to be no more and no less of a problem than it was a decade ago. There is an obvious need for new sound data.

THE CHANGING CONTENT OF PORNOGRAPHY

Present day advocates of greater legal control claim that there is now an overwhelming fusion of violence and pornography (Steinem, 1980; Brownmiller, 1975; Rush, 1980; Eysenck and Nias, 1978; Clue, 1974). Some critics of the Commission on Pornography claim that it failed to address this issue even though it was familiar with the work and conclusions of a similar Commission on Violence three years earlier. The Violence Commission had gathered data which clearly demonstrated that exposure to the pictorial portrayal of violence in the media led to increased aggressive behavior in the observers. The Pornography Commission was indeed aware of the conclusions of the Violence Commission and frequently discussed the disparity between the findings of the two Commissions. No conclusion could be reached except that the sexual stimulus apparently was different and weaker than the violent stimulus for transfer into anti-social and criminal behavior. Exposure to violence stimulated aggression but stimulation of sexual behavior was not noted. Similarly, exposure to pornography stimulated sexual behavior somewhat but effects on aggressive behavior were not noted. As for the fusion of violence and pornography, the Commission did not do a systematic study of the content of pornographic materials available in 1970. Its task was to focus on the explicit sexual content rather than on the context in which this was presented. Among the thousands of photos in magazines and the hundreds of motion pictures examined there is little doubt that the vast bulk of material consisted of trite and silly plots with the usual sexual acrobatics and the exhibition of genitalia in action taken with a close-up lens. There was very rarely bestiality, pedophilia, or violence. These were considered to be rare freaks in an already peculiar industry. The Commissioners and the staff themselves became sated and may have lost their sensitivity to the exhibition of combined sex and violence. Whatever the reason, it was insensitive and failed to address the problem of combined violence and erotica and its potential effects.

There is evidence that this has changed. The amount of pictorial non-sexual violence of all sorts in television and the movies has gone up substantially. The amount of violent crime in the nation continues to rise. The correlation between the two is significant and may or may not imply a causal connection. Such a connection is suggested by the large number of experimental findings that exposure to written or pictorial violence increases aggressive behavior to others during and after the experiment (Baron, 1977; Berkowitz, 1962). This should be a matter of considerable concern to law enforcement officials, behavioral scientists, teachers, and parents.

The fusion of pornography and violence is also stated to have increased, although the degree to which this has happened is difficult to assess because the Commission on Pornography failed to establish an adequate data base for the period prior to 1970.

Eysenck and Nias noted significant combinations of the two in 1978. Malamuth and Spinner (1980) analyzed pictorials and cartoons in *Playboy* and *Penthouse* from 1973 to 1977 and found an increase over this period, so that in 1977 about ten percent of the cartoons and 5 percent of the pictorials depicted sexual violence. Most of those were in *Penthouse*. If these data are projected back to the period 1960–1970 they would confirm the Commission impression that very little violent pornography was available at that time. The Malamuth and Spinner (1980) data show that the absolute level in this type of magazine is still very low. Smith (1976) examined 428 "adult" paperback novels and found 4588 explicit sexual episodes, of which approximately 195 involved rape. *Hustler* magazine, published ostensibly for the hard-hat, cigar smoking, beer drinker rather than the effete *Playboy* reader, had cartoons of a child molester until 1978 and still publishes letters (fictitious?) from women readers who express joy in masochistic domination and incest. "Variations," published by *Penthouse* ostensibly to spice diminishing sexuality, frequently alludes to bondage and other sadomasochistic variations as being pleasurable for both partners. Lederer (1980) states that a group of researchers from Women Against Violence in Pornography and Media (WAVPM) viewed 26 pornographic films in San Francisco. Twenty-one contained rape scenes, 16 had bondage and torture scenes, two featured killing of women for sexual stimulation, and two were films of child molestation. These figures are alarming if true. (WAVPM is militantly biased and such studies require replication by more objective observers.) A cursory examination of newspaper advertisements for X-rated films in many areas does not indicate by title if such films are more violent toward women. Their content may be.

Pornographers, it should be noted, are clever. The Pornography Commission report was quickly reprinted with 300 pornographic pictures added by a publisher who claimed that they were educational, illustrating the type of materials with which the Commission was concerned. The social response was notable. Reputable bookstores refused to merchandise it. The legal response was also clear; the publisher was tried and convicted of using the mails for distribution. A pornographic film the author saw a few years ago dealt with a virgin engaged to be married. In her premarital nightmares she dreamt of incest, gang rape, and bondage, all of which were explicitly presented on film. Her concerned parents sought a psychiatrist for her, leaving her overnight in the care of her boyfriend. This time her nightmares included sleepwalking to his bed. They made tender, explicit love with all types of pleasurable variations. When her parents returned she no longer needed psychiatric care and smilingly asked them to permit her to marry more quickly. Is this a fusion of pornography and violence? A comic morality play with loving sex triumphant? A fairy tale like Little Red Riding Hood, or a caricature of psychiatry? Should it be banned?

An imaginary script which should simultaneously please and offend everyone has been conjured up by the author. Imagine the following scenario for an X-rated movie:

Open with a lovely wedding in which there is a furtive angry man lurking in the audience. He follows the honeymooners on their honeymoon and acts as a "Peeping Tom" while they make explicit, ardent, and varied love. The next morning, while the husband jogs, the man breaks in, threatens the woman with a knife, and then has her perform fellatio with a knife at her throat. This is followed by some vulgar sexual acrobatics in which he constantly abuses and threatens her, meanwhile repeating that this is what women really like. To save herself, she pretends enjoyment which she acts out well enough to fool the rapist (and audience). It is so good a performance that she asks him back the next day. Her real disgust and fear are revealed only when her husband returns. To reassure her they again make ardent and endearing love. They also plot to capture the rapist the next day. Repeat the first orgy scene but this time have the husband interrupt. There is a bloody fight in which the husband is knifed. The naked wife saves him and the situation by knocking the rapist out with a vase. She ties him up, then cleanses and binds her husband's wounds, kisses and caresses him with vigor, and again they make ardent and varied love. They then revive the bound rapist, put him in a chair and discuss what to do with him. They decide to frighten and humiliate him. With the knife they threaten to gouge his eyes, slit his nose, mark and label him, or castrate him. She teasingly does that with manual manipulation of his penis and testicles while gesturing with the knife and verbally insulting him. Finally they punish him by putting a wastebasket over his head so that he can't see as they again make ardent love while uttering insults and contemptuous remarks to the rapist. They then dress, call the police, and are happily drinking coffee while he is taken away.

Moralists would be offended by all of the explicit sex but might be pleased by the triumph of law and order. Women might be pleased by the loving sex, offended by the rape, and pleased again by the types of punishment which the rapist receives. Even the most chauvinistic male who might enjoy almost everything else might be offended by the castration threat and humiliation of the rapist. Regardless of the legal tangles such a movie could generate, the producer would be concerned most with the old theatrical question. Would it play big in Peoria? It appears doubtful because the threatened castration scenes would be upsetting to the majority of the customers, who are men.

THE EFFECTS OF PORNOGRAPHY AND VIOLENCE

Many experiments have been conducted by psychologists in the past five years to examine the effects of exposure to erotica on aggression, and the effects of combined erotica and violence on aggression (Baron, 1977; Berkowitz, Donnerstein et al., 1975; Malamuth et al., 1977; White, 1980; Donnerstein, 1980; Fenigstein, 1979). The results indicate a complex relationship. Exposure to nonviolent erotica may inhibit, fail to affect, or facilitate aggression. Baron and Bell (1977) exposed 85 undergraduate males to pictures and paragraphs ranging from neutral to highly erotic.

Prior to the exposure they were angered or treated neutrally by a male confederate of the experimenters, and after the visual stimuli were permitted to aggress against this person by means of electric shock. The results showed that in both angered and nonangered subjects, exposure to mild erotica (bikinis, lingerie, and nude women) reduced later aggression by the male subjects to the confederate. Exposure to pictures of actual intercourse further diminished the aggressive response but exposure to erotic written passages restored the aggressive response to the level found with neutral stimuli. Under no conditions did exposure to erotica increase aggression above that found with neutral stimuli. This finding differs from that of other investigators (Zillman, 1971; Jaffe et al., 1974).

Jaffe et al. (1974) on the other hand found that exposure to erotica increased aggression. Baron and Bell (1977) suggest that the difference between their results and those of others may be due to the possibility that their most erotic stimuli were less arousing than that of the others. For example, they used still pictures, others used movies. In a later study using women subjects, Baron found that the same explicit sexual stimuli which inhibited aggression in male subjects increased it in female subjects. This may be because while both found it arousing, men judged the stimuli to be pleasant while women found it to be disgusting.

L. A. White (1980) exposed male college students to stimuli which were high or low in producing positive or negative effects. For the same level of sexual arousal, high negative response was produced by the same sex masturbation or highly explicit cunnilingus; positive effects by heterosexual fondling, intercourse, or fellatio. The subjects were also angered or not angered by confederates and were then able to respond aggressively to the confederates by shocking them. A control group was used that was angered but not exposed to any of the pictorial stimuli. The results showed that exposure to positive erotic stimuli reduced aggressive retaliatory behavior to a level below the control group. On the other hand, exposure to unpleasant or disgusting erotic stimuli enhanced subsequent aggressive behavior. White suggests that individuals who have difficulty controlling their anger might be taught to construct pleasant images as a means of reducing the intensity of their retaliatory responses.

Donnerstein (1980), who has studied the effects of erotic stimuli on aggressive behavior for several years, first noted that mild erotica inhibited aggression while highly erotic stimuli maintained aggression at a level similar to nonerotic exposure (Donnerstein et al., 1975). More recently, he has studied the effect of erotica on aggression against women. In his most recent work (1980), Donnerstein exposed 120 undergraduate males to sexually aggressive films and studied the effect of these stimuli on aggression towards both men and women. Both angered and nonangered men were employed as subjects. The nonaggressive sexual film showed a couple having intercourse; the aggressive one showed a woman being raped by a man with a gun.

The results showed that both the nonaggressive and aggressive film increased aggression toward males to a similar degree above the neutral stimulus. Aggression toward a woman was not increased by the simple erotic film, but was increased by the aggressive erotic film. When the subjects were previously angered, the erotic film produced a more aggressive response than the neutral film and the aggressive erotic film was associated with generating even more of an aggressive response. Thus, the optimum conditions for eliciting aggressive behavior involve first making the subject angry and then exposing him to an aggressive erotic film in which there is a woman victim. Under these experimental conditions, there is an increase in aggressive behavior toward men, but even more so toward women.

What can one determine from the types of experiments cited above? First, there is by now evidence that exposure of men to aggressive erotica enhances aggressive behavior to men and even more so to women. This is especially true when the men are angered prior to the experiment. The effects, though statistically significant, were not large, but nonetheless they may be indicative of what might happen to a much larger extent in real life situations. Thus, a man made furious by a woman in real life might view an aggressive-erotic film and then act out violently, especially toward a woman. On the other hand, angered men viewing a nonaggressive erotic film might find their anger and aggressive behavior diminished.

CONCLUSIONS

Despite what seem to be exaggerated claims, there is now evidence that some pornography is violent and that under some conditions the fusion of pornography and violence does lead to increased aggression toward men and more so toward women. I am therefore inclined to agree with Eysenck (1978), who says,

It seems clear to us that there are certain areas of sexual behavior which should be completely excluded from the list of permitted activities (for depiction on film); sex involving children is one such area; rape and other forms of sexual violence, vividly and explicitly presented, are others. Sex involving animals would probably also come into this category . . . Torture, bondage, and sadomasochistic acts involving sex may also be mentioned here. Such films may perhaps be shown on psychiatric prescription to patients addicted to such perversions, but they are not safe for public showing.

Incest should be added. Carrying out such limited censorship should be simpler than the existing problems of legally defining pornography because specific types of activities which can readily be defined are forbidden. The display of other types of sexual activity seems to be harmless and for consenting adults need not be governed by legal control. But such limited censorship will displease both those who feel it is too little and those who think it is too much. I would hope that more restrictive legislation would not be imposed until sound research has been conducted to demonstrate a need for it. Such research is not likely to be forthcoming in the near future because of the massive cuts in federally supported social and behavioral research. In the meantime, there is much to be admired in the statement of Wendy Kaminer (1980), an attorney who is a member of Women Against Pornography and who helped to draft their position paper on freedom of speech and pornography. She says,

Legislative or judicial control of pornography is simply not possible without breaking down the legal principles and procedures that are essential to our own right to speak and, ultimately, our freedom to control our own lives. We must continue to organize against pornography and the degradation of women, but we must not ask the government to take up our struggle for us. The power it will assume to do so will be far more dangerous to us all than the 'power' of pornography.

REFERENCES

Baron R: *Human Aggression.* New York, Plenum Press, 1977.
Baron RA, Bell PA: Sexual arousal and aggression by males: Effects of type of stimuli and prior provocation. *J Pers Soc Psychol* 35(2):79–87, 1977
Barry K: Beyond pornography: From poetics to creating a vision, in Lederer L (ed): *Take Back the Night:* New York, William Morrow & Co, 1980, pp 307–312
Brownmiller S: *Against Our Will: Men, Women, and Rape.* New York, Simon & Schuster, 1975

Clue V: *Where Do You Draw the Line?* Provo, Utah, Brigham Young University Press, 1974

Donnerstein E: Aggressive erotica and violence against women. *J Pers Soc Psychol* 39:269–278, 1980

Donnerstein E, Donnerstein M, Evans R: Erotic stimuli and aggression: Facilitation or inhibition? *J Pers Soc Psychol* 32:237–244, 1975

Eysenck N, Nias DKB: *Sex, Violence and the Media.* New York; St. Martin's Press, 1978

Fenigstein A: Does aggression cause a preference for viewing media violence? *J Pers Soc Psychol* 37:2307–2317, 1979

Gever M, Hall M: Fighting pornography, in Lederer L (ed): *Take Back the Night.* New York, William Morrow & Co, 1980, pp 279

Jaffe Y, Malamuth H, Feingold J, Feshbach S: Sexual arousal and behavioral aggression. *J Pers Soc Psychol* 30:759–764, 1974

Kaminer W: Pornography and the First Amendment: Prior restraints and private action, in Lederer L (ed): *Take Back the Night.* New York, William Morrow & Co, 1980, p 241

LaBelle B: Snuff-The ultimate in women hating, in Lederer L (ed: *Take Back the Night.* New York, William Morrow & Co, 1980, pp 272

Lederer L (ed): *Take Back the Night.* New York, William Morrow & Co, 1980

Lipton MA: Pornography, in Saddock B, Kaplon H, Freidman A (eds): *The Sexual Experience.* Baltimore, Williams & Wilkins Co, 1976, pp 584–594

Malmamuth NM, Feshbach S, Jaffe Y: Sexual arousal and aggression—recent experiments and theoretical issues. *J Soc Issues* 33:110–133, 1977

Malamuth N, Spinner B: A longitudinal content analysis of sexual violence in the best selling erotic magazines. *Journal Sex Res* August 1980

The Report of the Commission on Obscenity and Pornography. Superintendent of Documents, US Government Printing Office, September 1970

Rush F: Child pornograpy, in Lederer L (ed): *Take Back the Night.* New York, William Morrow & Co, 1980, p 80

Smith D: Sexual aggression in American pornography: The stereotype of rape. Presented to the American Sociological Association, New York City, 1976

Steinem G: Erotica and pornography: A clear and present difference, in Lederer L (ed): *Take Back the Night.* New York, William Morrow & Co, 1980, pp 35–40

White LA: Erotica and aggression: The influence of sexual arousal, positive affect and negative affect on aggressive behavior. *J Pers Soc Psychol* 37:269–278, 1980

Zillman D: Excitation transfer in communication—mediated aggressive behavior. *J Exp Soc Psych* 7:419–434, 1971

9

Alcoholism and Sexual Dysfunction

Laurence Schweitzer, Eleanor Brown, and Charles Tirrell

INTRODUCTION

Ethyl alcohol has a long, if only anecdotal, reputation as an aphrodisiac, sexual supporter, and improver of performance. The actual evidence for the role of alcohol in facilitating sexual activity is meager; that which has been collected supports the oft quoted Shakespearean view that it provokes the desire but takes away the performance. In this presentation we will attempt to review the biological and psychological effects of alcohol on human sexual functioning. We shall also attempt to draw out a set of theoretical speculations that bridge the biological and psychological aspects of this subject, and suggest some needed lines of research.

ENDOCRINE AND BIOCHEMICAL FACTORS

We begin with a consideration of endocrine factors, for it is here that our sexuality begins, develops, and is maintained. While we are aware of the role that sex steroids play in utero in organizing the ontogeny of the embryonal sex organs, we have been unable to document a related developmental anomaly associated with alcohol use during pregnancy. As alcoholism is still considered a disease of adults, we shall confine our comments to this age group although we recognize that sexuality is certainly not nearly so restricted. Finally, we make mention of the fact that the majority of the studies have focused on males, presumably because early data suggested that alcoholism affects males generally in a ratio of 5 to 1, that males' sexual functioning is more easily measured, and that most investigators have been men. Where possible we shall note the effects of alcohol on female sexual functioning.

As early as 1909, Kryle noted that testicular atrophy occurred in men with advanced liver disease. As most of his patients were alcoholics, he ascribed the loss of testicular volume to a direct toxic effect of the alcohol. This observation, as well as similar findings by Weichselbaum in 1911, went unnoticed for over a decade (Weichselbaum, 1911). During the mid-1920's Italian hepatologists again noted that alcohol-induced liver disease in males was associated not only with testicular atrophy, but with abnormal testicular histology, seminal fluid deficits, a female escutcheon, gynecomastia, and decreased libido and potentia. These latter two observations appear regularly in the literature, but nowhere is a description of these deficits available. The association of testicular atrophy, gynecomastia, and Laennec's cirrhosis was so well appreciated, however, that this symptom triad was accorded the eponym of Silvestrini-Corda syndome (Corda, 1939). No further attention was accorded to libido or potentia.

Almost two decades later, Reibler distinguished feminization from hypogonadism and speculated that feminization resulted from an accumulation of estrogenic substances in the plasma of cirrhotic men (Reibler, 1936). Since the liver was known to be intimately involved with the catabolism of sex hormones, it was assumed that a deficit in hepatic activity led to the retention of unconjugated estrogens. Further, it was generally accepted that postulated excess of estrogens led to suppression of pituitary gonadotrophin activity and thereby to decreased testicular activity and lowered androgen levels. Thus, the presumed role of alcohol shifted from that of a direct gonadal toxin to one of an indirect mode of activity by way of suppressing pituitary gonadotrophic activity (Bean, 1942). More recently, alcohol has again been ascribed the role of a direct toxin, causing injury to the hypothalamic-pituitary-gonadal axis with resulting failure of the anterior pituitary to release both follicle-stimulating hormone (FSH) and luteinizing hormone (LH) (Van Thiel and Lester, 1978).

Briefly, it is known that luteinizing hormone releasing hormone (LHRH) arises in the medial basal (median eminence) hypothalamic region and is transported by way of the portal circulation to the anterior pituitary where it causes LH and FSH to be released. The activity of

LHRH is, in turn, regulated by plasma testosterone levels and appears to be inhibited not only by the increased concentration of testosterone, but by estrogens as well. Thus, inhibition of LHRH can result in decreased release of LH and FSH with a consequent decrease in Leydig cell production of testosterone and, a secondary decrease of spermatogenesis (Van Thiel and Lester, 1976)

Gordon et al. (1976) studied the effect of chronic ethanol administration on normal males. They found that alcohol dampened the normal episodic bursts of testosterone secretion and was followed by a fall in the plasma level of the steroid during the first five days of alcoholization. Additional decreases in testosterone levels occurred when alcoholization continued for 12–14 days.

In 1978 Mendelson et al. repeated a similar study, this time using male alcohol addicts, and, more recently, reported a third replication with normal alcoholized males. In summary, it was found that testosterone levels decreased during the ascending portion of the blood alcohol concentration (BAC) curve with a further decrease in the concentration of testosterone at the peak BAC. During the ascending portion of the curve no change occurred in luteinizing hormone levels, but later at the peak BAC, LH levels were noted to increase. The succession of testosterone decrease and subsequent LH increases suggested that alcohol produced its major effect in a peripheral manner, that is by way of a direct toxic effect on the testis.

Similarly, Gordon, Southern, and Lieber found that the chronic administration of alcohol not only decreased pulsatile testosterone release initially, but later decreased testosterone and LH (Gordon et al., 1978). Thus, peripheral as well as central effects of alcohol appeared present. In addition, these studies, and many more recent ones, demonstrated that the observed changes in testicular volume and architecture as well as gonadotrophin levels were uncorrelated to the presence of liver damage or cirrhosis.

Mendelson et al. (1978) also demonstrated that in physiological doses alcohol decreased testosterone production in decapsulated testis and this occurred in a dose dependent manner. On the basis of these findings, the authors suggested that decreased testosterone levels and subsequent increases in luteinizing hormones may act to produce an alteration in sexual and aggressive drive states. The often reported sexual arousal in males while intoxicated and the compromise in performance may be consistent with the decreased testosterone and later increased LH levels. By way of contrast, opiates act to decrease LH levels first and secondarily produce decreases in testosterone. Behaviorally, it is also known that opiates tend to decrease both aggression and sexual behavior during intoxication (Mirin et al., 1976).

Finally, in support of the role of alcohol as a gonadal toxicant the following evidence can be cited. There is known alcohol dehydrogenase activity in the testis, which, during periods of intoxication, produces an excess of NADH (Van Thiel et al., 1974). As the oxidation of ethanol increases the relative proportion of NADH to NAD, NAD dependent enzymes involved in testicular steroidogenesis such as delta 5, delta 3 isomerase and 3-β-hydroxy steroid reductase, will be reduced in efficiency. Moreover, increased NADH levels may disrupt carbohydrate metabolism and testosterone synthesis in Leydig cells (Lieber, 1968). Finally, it is known that vitamin A is necessary for spermatogenesis (Van Thiel et al., 1974). Vitamin A is absorbed as the alcohol retinol, esterified in the gut, stored in the liver, and released upon demand. Retinol is oxidized to retinal within the testicle by alcohol dehydrogenase. However, alcohol dehydrogenase of the testicle has a 50 times greater affinity for ethanol than retinol and chronic consumption of alcohol competitively inhibits retinol transformation with the production of germ cell aplasia through a chronic deficiency of vitamin A (Van Thiel et al., 1974).

In contrast to the studies cited for males, there is a paucity of data concerning the endocrinological effects of alcohol in females. Wright et al. (1976) examined 13 alcoholic women and found elevated LH responses to LHRH. Similarly, McNamee et al. (1979) also failed to demonstrate a hypothalamic-pituitary-gonadal axis dysfunction in a study of eight actively alcoholic females. These limited data may also be taken to support the notion that alcohol exerts its major effect at the level of the gonads.

In summary, alcohol appears to disturb the normal hormonal balance of the gonadotrophins and sex steroids. Its mechanism of action is likely due to a direct inhibitory effect on the gonads and probably on the hypothalamic pituitary system as well. The previously advocated role of liver disease in producing these changes appears less important in light of newer biochemical findings and, indeed, some of the feminization features such as gynecomastia can now be related to a chronic elevation of serum prolactin in susceptible alcoholic males (Van Thiel et al., 1975).

Although the role of alcohol in altering hormone levels now appears well established, it is difficult to predict the effect that these changes produce on established patterns of sexual activity. There is less difficulty, however, in asserting that alcohol is a rapidly acting drug that has an acute major effect, the suppression of activity in higher cortical centers with concomitant changes in reaction time, judgment, and coordinated complex performance. Thus, it is of interest to study the acute and chronic physiological and psychological changes produced by alcohol on sexual activity.

PHYSIOLOGICAL CHANGES

Again, the number of physiological studies is very limited and largely restricted to acute effects seen in males. Moreover, most studies are seriously flawed since they have only examined the effects of alcohol on normal subjects. Nevertheless, the consistency of the findings prompts us to review and summarize these data as well as the limited findings in humans.

Gantt was among the first to examine the effects of alcohol on sexual performance (Gantt, 1952). Using dogs, he administered three doses of alcohol, 0.5 cc, 1.0 cc, and 2.0 cc/kg body weight, obtaining blood levels comparable to intoxicating conditions in humans. The results indicated that ejaculation was delayed and latency to tumescence lengthened in proportion to the dose. Hart (1968) also reported similar results in dogs although he used much higher doses of alcohol (4.0 cc/kg body weight). Hart's data most notably demonstrated that sexual motivation as measured by mountings persisted, although the dogs were markedly ataxic. The findings are similar in rats, except for a decrease in latency to first mount, intromission, and ejaculation (Hart, 1969). In general, the animal data support the notion of increased desire and decreased performance.

An extrapolation of these data suggests that alcohol would compromise erectile functioning in humans as well. It is likely that alcohol would also interfere with the willed inhibition of sexual responses to overt erotic and fantasized stimuli in humans since it is a cortical depressant. Rubin and Henson tested this hypothesis in a carefully designed study using 16 adult nonalcoholic males as subjects (Rubin, 1976). Explicit erotic material was presented via a television monitor during three experimental sessions. The first and third sessions were conducted under placebo conditions. In one half of the subjects the second session was carried out under three conditions of alcoholization that ultimately produced BAC of .1 to .15 mg percent.

Measures of sexual arousal included the maximum attained erection, the mean erection, and the latency to 20 percent of a full erection. With respect to arousal, the data were clear-cut. When BAC approximated .10 to .15 mg percent, a level generally accepted as intoxicating in nontolerant subjects, peak erections dropped to 40 percent of maximum. Mean erections generally decreased in proportion to the dose, and latency to 20 percent full erection was not significantly affected until after the last drink, when the mean time doubled. These data on arousal accord with the cited animal studies and the derived predictions, but the data regarding ability to inhibit sexual responses is more difficult to interpret.

In general, by the second drink, mean tumescence was decreased to some degree in over 70 percent of the subjects, but the degree of inhibition was small. The maximum attained erection was not influenced by the inhibition command and more than 50 percent of the subjects experienced larger peak erections and 73 percent more mean tumescence when instructed to inhibit arousal than during the baseline conditions. This appears to suggest that moderate alcohol use impairs the ability to inhibit arousal. In a similar study of normal controls, Farkas and Rosen also found that low doses of ethanol facilitated maximum tumescence, whereas higher doses drastically reduced penile diameter and tumescense rate (Farkas and Rosen, 1976).

While these data derived from nonalcoholic subjects are in line with the anecdotal and expected responses, alcoholics do not drink moderately and are tolerant to substantially larger doses of alcohol than normal volunteers. Thus it is impossible to predict the acute effects of alcohol in alcoholics from these laboratory studies.

We are unaware of any studies in which alcoholics have been exposed to physiological levels of alcohol and examined in similar fashion. There is one study of a more clinical nature, however, that does bear on the issue of erectile potency in alcoholics and these data will be briefly summarized.

Karacan et al. (1980) reported the results of a study of six alcoholics who were referred for sleep studies as part of a pre-surgical evaluation of implanting a penile prosthesis. As a direct measure of a patient's degree of impotence, the authors used nocturnal penile tumescence (NPT) as the pertinent variable. This small sample was obviously highly skewed as patients were selected for erectile impotence as well as their desire to change their symptom. It is unlikely that they were representative of alcoholics in general.

When compared to appropriate controls, these alcoholics displayed significantly fewer full erections (both in minutes and in number) and more partial NPT. Moreover, the peak erections attained tended to be reduced, suggesting a maintenance of tumescence but a decrease in a degree to which it is obtained in alcoholics.

Closer examination of the patients' reactions revealed that three of the alcoholics failed to ever achieve full NPT although they had exaggerated amounts of partial NPT. The remaining three patients did exhibit some episodes of full NPT, but the total duration was on the average 20 minutes less than controls. This latter group was regarded as physiologically sound but similar to other men complaining of impotence. The three who failed to ever achieve full NPT were, on the other hand, identified as having an organic deficit in the mechanism that allows for maximal engorgement of the penis. Thus, one half of the alcoholics complaining of impotence had physiological changes in their erectile mechanisms. Obviously, more study is needed on the correlation of long-term changes in these parameters to patterns of alcohol ingestion.

Data bearing on alcoholic female dysfunction is regrettably even more difficult to obtain. Viamontes anecdotally reports that some of his female patients complained of poor sexual desire, poor performance, and the absence of orgasm (Viamontes, 1974). No further descriptive information is provided on the question of performance during alcohol-abstinent periods. These subjective data would be relatively easy to obtain although the validity of the results would have to be viewed with some caution. For example, subjects alcoholized in the Rubin and Henson study regularly reported that they experienced an improvement in performance whereas objective measures of tumescence were quite the opposite.

PSYCHOLOGICAL-BEHAVIORAL FINDINGS

The previous data have dealt with the effects of alcohol on sexual activity, but the problem is doubly complicated. One must also consider the role of sexual conflicts as a motivational factor in the drinking behavior of nondependent subjects. The unravelling of psychosexual conflicts from the magnifying effects of alcohol is an extremely complex task. In this regard, one special value of sleep NPT studies is that it may avoid the issues of unconscious conflicts and motivational systems. However, a price must be paid for clean data and in this case it is the loss of ability to evaluate the complex interactions of psychology and pharmacology since the data will not relate to normal conscious experience.

Levine carried out an interesting study of the psychopathology of alcoholic patients who had received psychotherapy at a state operated outpatient clinic (Leoine, 1955). He used data from 79 of 400 patients treated during a six-month period and cases were selected on the basis of the completeness of the clinical record. The sample was rather representative of alcoholics in general, as there were four times as many males with an age range of 22–51 years. Unfortunately there was no description of the duration, intensity, or continuity of the drinking. There were no criteria supplied to evaluate if the subjects were alcohol abusers, the degree of tolerance attained, and the presence or absence of dependence. These very serious methodological flaws are underscored in the hope that we make more of an effort to document these parameters in future studies. Indeed, we have found that where attention has been paid to a description of the alcoholic behavior, only the crudest description of sexuality is provided, and where sexuality is well described, practically no attention is paid to the parameters of the alcoholism. The following surprising results must then be tempered by the fact that we cannot correlate Levine's sexual observations to the patients' degree of alcoholism. Finally, although the demographics of the sample are representative of alcoholics in general, the patients in this study were selected on the basis of other psychological problems and none were reported as seeking treatment for a sexual disturbance.

Levine (1955) found that 70 percent of the men reported sexual intercourse not more than once every three months, with 12 denying all sexual activity and 16 restricted to one to two times a year. The remaining 30 percent reported sexual activity as frequently as one to two times per week. There were also 16 women in the study, five of whom were described as promiscuous but also almost completely unable to achieve orgasm. Fifty percent of the women denied heterosexual activity at all; one was a virgin and the remaining seven said that they had no interest (Levine, 1955).

The expressed attitudes of these patients were quoted and it was very clearly documented that the alcoholic subjects were not interested in heterosexual relations. The most common factor was simply that sex was unimportant, and in this group, alcohol appeared to dissipate thoughts of sex. For example, one patient said "I never go in for that sort of stuff. Whenever I feel like that, I go someplace to get drunk. When I drink I never think about those things." Another male stated "I don't care much for girls. I would rather be with fellows. I have intercourse once in awhile—I have had it about 35 times in my life. I like to come and go as I please," or "Sex is a pretty minor matter with me because I can get along without having sex whatsoever." Among the women some comments were, "I have never had any interest in sex; I have never had an orgasm," or "I have no sexual feelings towards men, in fact, I don't like to have anything to do with sex. I never become aroused sexually." (Levine; 1955).

A more careful examination of the male responses suggested that they actually preferred males to females, whereas the females appeared to express a fear of men or hostile attitudes towards them. Thus, in general, chronic alcohol use was associated with a lowered interest in sex but it was not clear what was cause or effect. Noteworthy was the fact that the sample included two active homosexuals, both of whom stated that they could carry out their homosexual activity only when drunk, never when sober (Levine, 1955).

The fact that alcohol tends to be a sexual excitant and impairs willed inhibition at low or moderate levels leads to a consideration of its role in acts of sexual paraphilia. The majority of studies of incest have emphasized the role of alcohol in the expression of this act. For example, Holder (1974), found that 79 percent of fathers who committed incestuous acts were alcoholic. Other authors have found 50–80 percent of the fathers to be alcoholic and have also noted that the sexual act was very often associated with a great deal of aggressive behavior.

Virkkunen reviewed 45 cases of incest in Finland looking for specific characteristics of alcoholic incest offenders (Virkkunen, 1974). He found that almost half (47 percent) were clearly alcoholic and that most were intoxicated at the time of the act. This was in clear contrast to nonalcoholic offenders. Moreover, the alcoholic offenders demonstrated more evidence of previous criminality, especially acts of violence. The data were interpreted as supporting the notion that alcohol had served to trigger the release of these perverse acts.

More recently, Browning and Boatman examined 14 cases of incest seen at the University of Oregon Hospital (Browning and Boatman, 1977). Again, alcohol use appeared to play a prominent role in the adults' behavior, as 8 of 14 were identified as either problem drinkers with severe psychopathology or as clear-cut alcoholics.

Finally, Rada has provided some very interesting data concerning the relationship of alcohol to child molestation (Rada, 1976). In a study of 203 child molesters he found that almost one half (49 percent) were drinking at the time of the offense and that a third (34 percent) were drinking heavily. Interestingly, a significantly greater percentage of the molesters were drinking when the sexual object was a girl. That is to say if the act included a homosexual object, it was less likely to be associated with alcohol use.

Aside from the dramatic association between alcoholism, alcohol use, and child molestation, it is interesting that pedophilic homosexual activity is associated to a lower rate of alcoholism as well as intoxication. One interpretation of these data consistent with the findings already reported is as follows: individuals with homosexual object choices would be likely to have a greater degree of internalized nonreactive pathology. They would also be likely to experience less impediment to acting on their pedophilic impulses than individuals whose normal sexual object was the opposite sex. In support of this idea, Virkkunen (1974) noted that the alcoholic pedophiliacs reported significantly greater rejection by their spouses and greater sexual frustration, a situation apparently caused by their drinking and their related poor socioeconomic conditions. Thus, alcohol use may have a significant effect in impairing sexual and aggressive inhibitions in individuals who by virtue of circumstance or emotional illness find their normal sexual outlets unavailable. The use of alcohol in such situations may induce some individuals to carry out deviant sexual behavior (Rada, 1975).

There is also a strong association between drinking, alcoholism, and rape. Johnson, Gibson, and Linder (1978) found that 72 percent of the rapes in Winnipeg, Canada occurred when one or more of the individuals had been drinking. Moreover, the likelihood of force being used was greater when alcohol was present, the relationship depending to some degree on who was drinking. The relationship was weakest when the victim alone was drinking, and greatest when both had been drinking. Although the authors of this study suggest that the circumstances of drinking produce greater changes in behavior than the alcohol use, the association of alcohol use, sexual deviation, and the expression of concomitant aggression is very striking.

The relationship of alcoholism and homosexuality is also well-known and will only be briefly noted here without suggesting either cause or effect. Both male and female homosexuals have far greater percentages of alcoholism than the general population (Saghir et al., 1970). In addition, very substantial proportions of homosexuals report that sexual activity occurs under the influence of intoxicating levels of alcohol and many find it a necessary precondition for satisfactory sexual activity.

Whether alcohol use produces stimulation of appetitive centers in the brain, decreases inhibitions, or occurs in social settings conducive to these actions, the association between alcohol and sexual deviation is one that obviously needs further clarification.

Aside from laboratory studies or epidemiological reviews, what do we know about the effects of alcohol on sexual performance from a clinical perspective? Unfortunately, very little. For example, Lemerer and Smith reported that of 17,000 patients treated for alcoholism, eight percent of the males complained of impotence (Lemerer and Smith, 1973). In 50 percent of the cases the potency problems persisted even after years of sobriety, prompting the authors to suggest that long-term injury to the autonomic innervation of the penis had occurred. They stressed the organic disturbance of erection since the majority of their patients reported a strong desire for sex. This anecdotal report was, of course, partially confirmed by the later results of Karacan, who found that 50 percent of the alcoholics presenting with erectile difficulties were unable to achieve a full nocturnal erection, a finding compatible with an organic dysfunction (Karacan, et al. 1980).

We have found only one other clinical report of sexual dysfunction, this time in women. In this case the subjects complained of delayed orgasm (Malatesta and Pollack, 1980). In contrast to the paucity of studies on alcoholism and sexual dysfunction, Masters and Johnson (1970) report that alcohol use is the second greatest cause of secondary sexual dysfunction. Clearly, there is a need for clinical studies of alcoholic populations with a focus on their sexual behavior, alcohol use, and the presence of tolerance and/or dependence.

How can these data be synthesized in a psychological context? Currently, the Diagnostic and Statistical Manual of Mental Disorders (DSM III) (1980) assigns the pathological use of alcohol to a category called substance use disorder. Specifically, there are two pathological states; the first of which we call alcohol abuse and the second, alcohol dependence. The remaining familiar alcohol-related diagnoses are now found as part of the organic mental disorders, in a subclassification called substance induced organic mental disorders.

Among many notable changes wrought by DSM III, alcoholism has been removed from the general category of character disorders. Yet, our definition of alcohol abuse continues to suggest a characterological quality. For example, the following, quoted from DSM III, suggests an impulse disorder: "There is a need for daily use for adequate functioning, an inability to cut down or stop drinking, and repeated efforts to control or reduce excess drinking by going on the wagon, etc." Later, elements of the definition suggest compulsive features: "Continuation of drinking despite serious physical disorders that the individual knows are exacerbated by alcohol use." The remaining criteria include impairment in social or occupational functioning and a duration of one month.

Based on these criteria, the alcoholic's behavior is obviously inflexible, maladaptive and causes significant impairment of social and vocational functioning. Yet these are the same general characteristics that DSM III uses to describe personality disorders and it seems reasonable, even if we do not classify it as such, to ascribe powerful personality or characterological features to alcohol abuse or dependence.

In this context it is interesting to recall that following World War I and World War II, there was a marked increase in the number of character disorders reportedly seen and, in particular, an increase in the treated addictions (DSM III, 1980). It has been speculated that the cessation of armed conflict deprives men of their psychological and physical participation in a larger entity and its laudable goals. The bitter fruit of victory or peace for the citizen is a return to individual social and economic responsibility. That is to say, individual social functioning requires renunciation of one's sexual and aggressive proclivities with the sublimation or derivative expression of these drives in appropriate and adaptive social activities. Without sublimation or derivative expression by way of participation in the aims of a larger group and its sanctions of sexual and aggressive behavior, the individual experiences what Freud termed "living beyond one's mental means." This feeling has further been described as a source of a feeling of discontent in our civilization. Examples of socially sanctioned activities that decrease our discontent would include organized gambling, athletic participation, sporting events, hunting, and a number of social organizations that have traditionally been exclusively male or female. Among the most important of these activities may be the socially responsible use of alcoholic beverages, as it participates in all of the preceding social institutions.

These abstract observations may now be brought to sharper focus if we recall the close association between alcohol use, alcoholism, and acts of sexual violence. Data derived from the molestation and rape studies suggest that alcohol use may, in some individuals, facilitate the expression of drive states that are generally strongly repressed and often excessively frustrated. In contrast, the more deviant forms of sexual and aggressive behavior would appear to be less well-controlled by intrapsychic forces and thus less dependent upon alcohol for facilitation or expression. In these cases the association to alcoholism and/or usage is weaker.

In 1948, Ernest Simmel proposed a classification of alcoholism that is relevant to this discussion. Simmel divided drinkers into social, reactive, and neurotic types, these categories corresponding to subtypes of the abuser. A fourth category, alcohol addict, corresponded to the alcohol dependent individual.

Social drinkers were described as those individuals who are chronically dependent upon moderate amounts of alcohol in order to enjoy their associations with other people. They cannot converse meaningfully with others or do business without drinking or offering a drink to those with whom they are dealing. Alcohol appears to help make these people congenial when they would be more likely to experience strong competitive strivings or would otherwise dislike each other because of the need to renounce or sublimate shared sexual and aggressive impulses. In many such cases the use of alcohol is most helpful and facilitates social intercourse. It is a clear example of society institutionalizing a practice that allows for the sublimation of conflicted impulses.

The reactive drinker is not necessarily neurotic either, for in this case the external circumstances of his personal life may impose too much deprivation. Instances of this situation include an unhappy marriage or work situation.

On the other hand, the neurotic drinker does not drink because of an insoluble entanglement with his environment, but rather to escape from his self-inflicted neurotic misery. For these people the business of living, loving, or working always has an unconscious connotation that brings their pursuit of happiness into conflict with their conscience. Trivial examples include men who begin drinking or who become impotent when their wives become pregnant or deliver a child. Often alcohol dissolves the taboo of taking a mother for one's sexual object, and facilitates adequate sexual functioning. In these cases, the judicious use of alcohol guarantees pleasure and often becomes a precondition for sexual performance.

In participating and mediating between a forbidden unconscious impulse and its expression, neurotic alcoholism appears to correspond to our older notion of a perversion. Indeed, the use of alcohol decreases anxiety while allowing for direct sexual gratification. Unfortunately, when alcohol becomes necessary for functioning, its pharmacological features begin to dominate the clinical picture. The development of tolerance requires more drug to relieve anxiety, but this condition ultimately produces more frustration as it is likely to increase desire while compromising performance. The net effect is for drinking to ultimately dominate one's life and for one to become progressively more preoccupied with the acquisition and availability of spirits. This preoccupation inevitably leads to isolation and a reduction of social contact. Often the preferred company becomes a group of one's own sex, wherein the group activity displaces direct sexual and aggressive drives through shared fantasy, discussion, or the breakthrough of primitive impulses.

Finally as a true dependent state occurs, that is, as an addictive state develops, we see a complete loss of control with frequent outbursts of aggressive behavior. Object relations disappear and are replaced by an attraction to and an overwhelming compulsion to obtain alcohol. While profound psycho-biological issues are at work by this time in the illness, the meaning of this behavior clearly indicates that the sought after, prized, and sexually cathected object, alcohol, is cannibalistically and suicidally consumed. Thus, while alcohol initially improves desire and perhaps prolongs sexual performance, its prolonged use decreases performance and destroys opportunities for normal sexual activity.

REFERENCES

Bean WB: A note on the development of cutaneous arterial spiders and palmar erythema in persons with liver disease and their development following administration of estrogens. *Am J Med Sci* 204: 251, 1942

Browning DH, and Boatman B: Incest: Children at risk. *Am J Psychiatry* 134: 69, 1977

Corda L: *Minerva Med* 5: 1067, 1925, cited by Edmonson HA, Class, SJ, Sol SN: Gynecomastia associated with cirrhosis of the liver. *Proc Soc Exp Biol Med* 42: 97–99, 1939

Diagnostic and Statistical Manual of Mental Disorders (DSM III). Washington, DC, American Psychiatric Association, 1980, p 163–179

Farkas GM, Rosen RC: Effect of alcohol on elicited male sexual response. *J Stud Alcohol* 37: 265, 1976

Gantt WH: Effect of alcohol on the sexual reflexes of normal and neurotic male dogs. *Psychosom Med* 14: 174, 1952

Gordon GG, Altman K, Southren AL, et al: Effect of alcohol (ethanol) administration on sex-hormone metabolism in normal men. *N Engl J Med* 295: 793, 1976

Gordon GG, Southren AL, Lieber CS: The effects of alcohol liver disease and alcohol ingestion on sex hormone levels. *Alcohol Clin Exp Res* 2: 259, 1978

Hart BL: Effects of alcohol on sexual reflexes and mating behavior in the male dog. *Q J Stud Alcohol* 29: 839, 1968

Hart BL: Effects of alcohol on sexual reflexes and mating behavior in the male rat. *Psychopharmacology* (Berlin) 14: 377, 1969

Holder H: in Virkkunen M: Incest offenses and alcoholism. *Med Sci Law* 14: 124, 1974

Johnson SD, Gibson L, Linden R: Alcohol and rape in Winnipeg, 1966–1975. *J Stud Alcohol* 39: 1887, 1978

Karacan I, Snyder S, Salis PJ, et al: Sexual dysfunction in male alcoholics and its objective evaluation, in Fann WE et al (eds): *Phenomenology and Treatment of Alcoholism*. New York, Spectrum Publications, 1980, p 259

Kyrle J: Ueber stucter momalien in menschlichen hodenparenchym. *Verhandl Deutsch Pathol Gesellsch* 13: 391, 1909

Lemere F, and Smith JW: Alcohol-induced sexual impotence. *Am J Psychiatry* 130: 212, 1973

Levine J: The sexual adjustment of alcoholics: A clinical study of a selected sample. *Q J Stud Alcohol* 16: 675, 1955

Lieber CS: Metabolic effects produced by alcohol in the liver and other tissues, in Stollerman GH (ed): *Advances in Internal Medicine,* vol 14. Chicago, Year Book Medical Publishers, 1968, pp 151–199

Malatesta VJ, Pollack R: Medical aspects of female sexuality. *Mod Med* 51: 50, 1980

Masters WH, Johnson VE: *Human Sexual Inadequacy.* Boston, Little Brown & Co, 1970

McNamee B, Grant J, Ratcliff J, et al: Lack of effect of alcohol on pituitary-gonadal hormones in women. *Br J Addict* 74: 316, 1979

Mendelson JH, Ellingboe J, Mello NK, and Kuehnle J: Effects of alcohol on plasma testosterone and luteinizing hormone levels. *Alcohol Clin Exp Res* 2: 255, 1978

Mirin SM, Mendelson JH, Ellingboe J, et al: Acute effects of heroin and naltrexone on testosterone and gonadotrophin secretion: A pilot study. *Psychoneuroendocrinology* 1: 359, 1976

Rada RT: Alcoholism and forcible rape. *Am J Psychiatry* 132: 444, 1975

Rada RT: Alcoholism and the child molester. *Ann NY Acad Sci* 273: 492, 1976

Reibler R: Ueber einen fall von gynokomastie und leberzirrhose. *Wein Klein Wochenschr* 49: 1076–1077, 1936

Rubin HB, Henson DE: Effects of alcohol on male sexual responding. *Psychopharmacology* 47: 123, 1976

Saghir MT, Robbins E, Walbran B, et al: Homosexuality. IV. Psychiatric disorders and disability in the female homosexual. *Am J Psychiatry* 127: 65, 1970

Simmel E: Alcoholism and Addiction. *Psychoanal Q* 17: 6, 1948

Van Thiel DH, Gavaler JS, Lester R: Ethanol inhibition of vitamin A metabolism in the testes: Possible mechanism for sterility in alcoholics. *Science* 186: 941, 1974

Van Thiel DH, Gavaler JS, Lester R, et al: Plasma estrone, prolactin, neurophysin and sex steroid-binding globulin in chronic alcoholic men. *Metabolism* 24: 1015, 1975

Van Thiel DH, Lester, R: Alcoholism: Its effect on hypothalamic-pituitary-gonodal function. *Gastroenterology* 71: 318, 1976

Van Thiel DH, Lester, R: Alcoholism: Its effect on hypothalamic-pituitary gonadal alcoholic men. *Alcohol Clin Exp Res* 2: 265, 1978

Viamontes JA: Alcohol abuse and sexual dysfunction. *Med Asp Hum Sex* 8: 185, 1974

Virkkunen M: Incest offenses and alcoholism. *Med Sci Law* 14: 124, 1974

Weichselbaum A: Ueber veranderunger der hoden bei chronischem alkoholismus. *Verhandl Deutsch Pathol Gesellsch* 14: 234, 1910

Wright JW, Fry DE, Merry J, Marks V: Abnormal hypothalamic-pituitary-gonadal function in chronic alcoholics. *Br J Addict* 71: 211, 1976

10

Abortion: Psychosexual Issues

Betsy S. Comstock

INTRODUCTION

Understanding the psychological implications of abortion would seem to be a major aspect of understanding both male and female adult functioning, considering the central place given to procreative functions in human development. In surveying the English language literature over the past 12 years, little reference was found to the impact of fetal loss for males. There was considerable attention paid to females with unwanted pregnancy in the decade from 1965 to 1975 when various English speaking nations were developing legislation legalizing voluntary termination of pregnancy. Most of the psychiatric literature focused on morbidity occasioned by unwanted pregnancy (Ford et al., 1972; Uddenberg, 1974; Drower and Nash, 1978a; Olley, 1970; Talan and Kimball, 1972; Patt et al., 1969; Fleck, 1970; Senay, 1970; Burkle, 1977), on follow-up studies after voluntary abortion (Drower and Nash, 1978a; Patt et al., 1969; Fleck, 1970; Senay, 1970; Kumar and Robson, 1978; Lipper and Feigenbaum, 1976; Warnes, 1971; Spaulding and Cavenar, 1978; Belsey et al., 1977; Corney and Hornton, 1974; Ewing and Rouse, 1973; Wallerstein et al., 1972; Brewer et al., 1977; Greenglass, 1976), and on comparisons of women terminating and women completing pregnancies (Ford, 1972; Kumar and Robson, 1978; Illsby and Hall, 1976; Drower and Nash, 1978b). Most researchers paid attention to pre-pregnancy psychiatric diagnoses (Uddenberg, 1974; Drower and Nash, 1978a; Olley, 1970; Burkle, 1977; Warnes, 1971; Belsey et al., 1977; Illsby and Hall, 1976;

Drower and Nash, 1978b), but very few published papers attempted to deal with the psychodynamic significance of abortion (Burkle, 1977; Warnes, 1971; Fischer, 1973; Deutsch, 1945).

It is the hypothesis of this paper that a better understanding of the significance of abortion can be obtained if attention is paid first to the types of abortion and their different effects on parents and if the impact of the various types of abortion is studied with respect to psychodynamic issues related to the developmental level of the parents. The discussion will be limited to the impact of abortion on women for no other reason than that there is a paucity of data from studies of males, either regarding the conscious or unconscious-symbolic meaning of pregnancy or regarding reactions to fetal loss.

LITERATURE REVIEW

Several extensive reviews are available in this area (Fleck, 1970; Illsby and Hall, 1976; Deutsch, 1945; Simon and Senturia, 1966; Abraham, 1969), probably the best being that by Illsby and Hall (1976) in the Bulletin of the World Health Organization. A comprehensive review will not be repeated here, but salient areas of concern will be identified.

A MEDLINE search of the English language literature on "Psychiatric Issues related to Abortion" revealed 582 citations in the past 12 years. Several changes related to the passage of time are important. The older literature tended to emphasize the deleterious effects of abortion (Rosen, 1954). In their 1966 review, Simon and Senturia identified the confusing diversity of results of outcome studies to that date. More recent literature has emphasized the relatively good outcome to be expected both from therapeutic and from voluntary abortion (Patt et al., 1969; Fleck, 1970; Senay, 1970; Belsey et al., 1977; Ewing and Rouse, 1973; Greenglass, 1976; Lane Commission Report, 1974).

The overall trend in psychiatric opinion toward more optimism about abortion parallels social and legal changes. In the US, medical abortion has shifted from being unusual on psychiatric indication, through an interval of liberalized legislation and interpretation of legislation, to being less remarkable in the current era of voluntary abortion. Issues of importance in the past have largely vanished: the stigmatization of abortion is reduced, and medical and psychiatric complications from illegal, nonmedical abortions have all but disappeared.

Epidemiologic studies of abortion have been plagued by methodological problems and by defects in research design. Reactions of not wanting a pregnancy must be very common. Kumar and Robson (1978) reported that in England in 1975 there were 138,000 legal abortions and 569,000 live births, that is, almost 20 percent of pregnancies were terminated by legal abortion. Fleck (1970) reported estimates in 1970 for the US that ten percent of pregnancies end in spontaneous abortion and over 25 percent in voluntary abortions, either legal or illegal. Uddenberg (1974) studied a random sample of young women in Sweden during their first pregnancy, and learned that 50 percent reported unplanned pregnancies and 38 percent reported either mixed feelings or negative feelings.

There is a tendency in the literature for generalizations from the most-studied groups to the total group of women who do not want their pregnancies. The most-studied groups are those referred to psychiatrists for abortions on psychiatric indications. The governing criteria for abortion vary from study to study, and biases based on moral judgments can be seen to influence these studies. A few general conclusions may be valid:

1. Post-abortion morbidity is highest in women who have serious pre-pregnancy psychopathology (Patt et al., 1969; Senay, 1970; Warnes, 1971; Belsey et al., 1977; Greenglass, 1976). However, Ewing and Rouse (1973) report a study in which this was not confirmed.

2. Post-abortion psychosis does not occur at a rate as high as that of post-partum psychosis (Fleck, 1970; Brewer, 1977). Even this finding is contradicted by at least one study (Jansson, 1965).

3. Spontaneous abortion does not seem to be associated with increased psychiatric symptoms in subsequent pregnancies but voluntary abortion is associated with a slightly increased rate of first trimester depression (Kumar and Robson, 1978).

4. Comparisons between women obtaining abortions and those refused abortion suggest greater morbidity in the latter groups (Drower and Nash, 1978b); to this morbidity must be added the pathogenesis of being unwanted for the child. Fleck (1970) states this dramatically, "Preventive psychiatry's single most effective tool is the prevention of unwanted offspring . . ."

To add to the difficulty of understanding the significance of abortion, the emergence of techniques for identifying fetal pathology in utero has created a new set of women qualifying for abortion because of the likelihood of producing a defective child (Jansson, 1965). The impact of what may be termed eugenic abortions has not been studied systematically. Amniocentesis for diagnosis of fetal abnormality is now commonplace, and no doubt in the future the psychiatric implications for this special group of women will be examined.

To date, psychoanalytic literature has focused on abortion remarkably infrequently. Freud (1955) recognized that unexpected morbidity may result after seemingly unambivalent decisions for abortion. Newell Fisher (1973) has presented a detailed case report of a woman compulsively repeating pregnancy and abortion whose motivation was considered alternating oedipal incestuous acting out and undoing. He cites V. Calif's similar formulation with respect to fantasies of infanticide.

TYPES OF ABORTION

Research has tended to focus on one or another type of abortion, without adequate attention directed to the different experiences related to different circumstances of fetal loss.

This paper will distinguish three types of abortion, with two subtypes, as follows:
1. Spontaneous abortion
2. Therapeutic abortion
   a. General medical indications
   b. Psychiatric indications
3. Voluntary abortion for unwanted pregnancy

In general, from a psychodynamic viewpoint, these types have in common the global reaction to fetal loss, which involves both the unconscious significance of conception and the mourning process following abortion. They differ in that spontaneous abortion usually is an unwanted experience, as may be therapeutic abortion. Therapeutic abortion for medical causes has implications of maternal or paternal incompetence and thus adds a sense of personal failure to the other stresses related to the pregnancy. Voluntary abortion is least likely to be associated with conflict except for those women and their families who experience uncertainty about the moral basis for fetal sacrifice, or when there is divided family opinion about the desirability of terminating the pregnancy.

THE UNCONSCIOUS MEANING OF PREGNANCY

Whatever their conscious reaction to pregnancy may be, women seem strongly affected by unconscious perceptions of the meaning of producing a baby. These perceptions vary with the woman's own level of psychosexual development. It must be emphasized that for any woman, psychosexual stage must be understood as the effort of the maturing individual to deal with needs and conflicts specific to sequential developmental periods. Difficulties at one stage may cause entry into the next stage with specific ego impairments, or may prohibit further maturation if ego impairment is sufficiently severe. Thus, as seen in the following examples, complex meanings of pregnancy may result as sequential conflicts are managed by sequential developmental compromise formations.

Pregnancy as Affirmation of Body-Self

An 18-year-old woman entered therapy with depressive symptoms and with a history of unstable relationships begun with distrust and terminated over seemingly trivial problems. There was a mildly autistic flavor in much of her thinking. She became pregnant out of wedlock and was delighted. She chose to have her baby, reporting that it gave her an identity, establishing for her a firm sense of being, clarity about sexual identity, and purpose in living.

Although this certainly could have been seen as the resolution of an adolescent identity crisis, it also related to the early life task of individuation and establishing ability to trust. The benefits in her life extended beyond the mother role, as she became more accepting of others and better able to function interpersonally.

Pregnancy as a Source of Oral Gratification

Many mothers acknowledge vicarious pleasure in their infants' obvious oral pleasure from sucking and satiation. A few mothers, themselves very dependent personalities, reveal their happy expectations of what their infant will give to them, usually expressed as companionship, understanding, and affection. Thus, the pregnancy is perceived as a means by which the mother will gain nurturant supplies.

Pregnancy as a Possession

The Roman noblewoman who said of her sons, "These are my jewels," was but one in a vast company of women for whom a major aspect of pregnancy is production and retention of something of value. Parenting issues of control and domination are conspicuous among these mothers so that they have emotional difficulty with the child's autonomous striving. Their prenatal fantasies center on the satisfaction of having someone over whom they will have full charge.

Pregnancy as a Solution for Envy of the Male

Although women today resent the central place given in the psychoanalytic psychology to penis envy, it still is true that women envy the power and greater social opportunites afforded men. At the anatomic level this is reflected in the satisfaction derived from the fact that men have impressive external genitalia but only women can have babies. The masculine advantage is a continuous one, whereas childbearing can only be intermittent and usually infrequent. It is my clinical impression that when envy of males is an important basis for conflict, women are especially apt to experience pregnancy as joyful and delivery as trouble-free. A high level of denial of the inevitable discomforts of pregnancy is necessary if the pregnancy is to be experienced as the validation of feminine power and attainment.

Pregnancy as Oedipal Triumph

Just as most girls in the age range of four to six years harbor some interest in growing up and marrying Daddy, so also many procreative women perceive their pregnancies as oedipal triumphs. The ideal situation of foregoing the infantile attachment to father, and substituting a nonincestuous partner, generally is accomplished in fact without complete disappearance of the unconscious wish for father's child.

These five unconscious meanings of pregnancy, and their various possible combinations, are observed clinically when there is substantial conflict related to them and in individuals who have developed inadequate defenses against the attendant conflicts.

INTRAPSYCHIC CONFLICT AND RELATED SYMPTOMS

For any unconscious meaning assigned to pregnancy, corresponding conflicts and symptoms can be enumerated, as shown in Table 1.

Although this tabulation is constructed from the starting place of a theoretical statement of developmental psychosexual conflicts, there is abundant clinical experience to document the occurrence of the various symptoms enumerated. Naturally many cases seen clinically overlap the categories separated for this tabulation. Psychodynamic issues rarely can be simply conceptualized.

PATIENT CARE ISSUES RELATED TO ABORTION

The existing literature provides little help for the psychiatrist in dealing with abortion-related issues since it contains so many conflicting findings. A central proposition in this paper is that much of the confusion results from the failure to separate types of abortion, and from failure to specify the level of personality organization of subjects studied.

Several clinical tasks face the psychiatrist. Providing evaluations and consultative opinions on the advisability of therapeutic abortion was common in the decade 1965–1975. This has changed since legislation has condoned voluntary termination of pregnancy. Should the Right to Life movement reverse this legislation, psychiatrists again will be asked to make judgements about whether the life or well-being of a pregnant woman is jeopardized by her pregnancy. Senay (1970) has provided lucid guidelines for these decisions. On the basis of personal experience with many such evaluations early in 1970, the following generalizations are added.

Substantial ambivalence about pregnancy signals major unconscious conflict of some kind. It seems unwise to support a recommendation for abortion until an evaluation has been done in sufficient depth to allow understanding of the woman's mixed feelings. There certainly are times when delivery of the baby may cause less associated morbidity than does abortion. Alternatives via adoption should be explored when women continue to feel ambivalent after the recommendation for abortion has been explored.

The prediction of suicide risk has been a central feature in decisions for therapeutic abortion on psychiatric indications. Prediction of suicide is at best a treacherous undertaking. The published frequency of suicide among pregnant women is sufficiently low to make prediction in a given case impossible by any techniques available now. In the past, suicidal thoughts were reported regularly by women seeking therapeutic abortion. Some, interviewed for follow-up studies, even admitted to having been coaxed by leading questions about suicidal thinking from the psychiatrists who evaluated them. Psychiatrists cannot reliably say that an individual will commit suicide because of a life-stress such as unwanted pregnancy. The most which can be said about those individuals with past history of suicide attempt, those with severe self-punishing depression, those with past history of poor impulse control, and those who verbalize feelings of hopelessness and frustration, is that some risk (statistically

TABLE 1. PREGNANCY MEANING, SYMPTOMS, AND REACTIONS TO ABORTION

Unconscious Meaning	Conflict	Symptoms Related to Pregnancy and Childbearing	Emotional Reactions to Abortion		
			1. Spontaneous	2. Therapeutic a. Medical b. Psychiatric	3. Voluntary
Affirmation of Body-Self	Fear of loss of pregnancy and thus loss of physical state as procreative woman	Fear of labor and delivery Perception of infant as extension of self with opposition to individuation Return to earlier somatic dysfunction after termination	Somatic dysfunctions secondary to loss of body-ego-reinforcement provided by pregnancy. Immediate grief reaction. Sexual identity confusion.		
Oral gratification	Fear of loss of nurturance expected in fantasied inverse relationship Reality experience of infant as helpless & needy	Failure to nurture; infant rejection Reaction-formation with overprotective responses	Anaclitic depression; sense of helplessness or relief from sadness		

Production and Retention	Autonomy conflict with need to control infant	Guilt over infant's "bad" behavior / Rigid mothering / Resistance to infant's autonomous functions / Possessiveness	Depression: sense of personal failure, self-blame / Increased obsessional symptoms if pregnancy ambivalence was severe	Variable reactions to "necessary abortion" with some self-blame	Rationalization Reaction-formation / Pleasure in "control of own destiny"
Affirmation of Feminine Power	Fear of "deprived" status as a woman	Over-investment in child production / Inability to share with mate	Disappointment, loss of self-esteem	Resignation, severe grief reaction if genetic defect in infant / Motivated abortion / Unlikely (Psych.)	Ambivalence in choosing abortion, thus subsequent grief likely, with self-blame
Oedipal Triumph	Incest taboo	Ambivalence about pregnancy with mixed pleasure and guilt / Abortion seeking	Relief from Oedipal guilt but with disappointment	Acceptance / Unlikely (Psych.)	As with spontaneous abortion, mixed feelings of relief and disappointment

low) exists for these people and that the risk is likely increased in those who state they contemplate suicide as a solution to crisis.

When patients are evaluated from the perspective of psychosexual conflict, little help is gained in risk prediction. Less well-defended, primitively organized personalities are more apt to make impulsive suicide efforts. However, better organized personalities may experience very intense guilt and may seek both relief and settling of scores via suicide. In general it is my impression that the degree of narcissistic pathology activated by a woman's pregnancy is the best indicator of suicide risk. Life threatening suicide risks among pregnant women usually are associated with experiencing the fetus as something foreign, not of the self, that violates body integrity, and threatens disfigurement, disability, or death.

Pregnancy is a life crisis for some women. The interpersonal aspects of this crisis have not been explored in this paper, which focuses on psychosexual conflict. Nevertheless, issues of family and institutional moral judgments and pressures from important others have major reality impact on the patient anticipating abortion. When patients feel determined to have their pregnancy terminated they use a great deal of denial about personal and family-group moral convictions. It should be the psychiatrist's responsibility to clarify these and to aid the patient in weighing immediate distress against possible long-term consequences of the decision for abortion. As in other crisis interventions, the psychiatrist brings to the situation of difficult decision making a better ability to perceive the time dimensions of a problem and to support the patient in projecting herself into future time.

Helping patients cope with the aftermath of abortion is an important additional task of the psychiatrist. While the necessity for this work is more readily recognized in situations of voluntary and therapeutic abortions, the aftermath of spontaneous abortions seems a remarkably neglected area. In the light of the various nuances of meaning associated with conception, the unexpected loss of a pregnancy is a deeply felt experience. Much depends on how real the anticipated baby has become for the expectant mother. Senay's (1970) suggestions for exploring fantasies about the baby are very helpful in this regard. When the baby has been cathected as an expected new person, a grief reaction will follow. Otherwise, the woman's emotional focus will be on her body-reproductive-failure or on her concern about having conceived a blighted fetus.

After induced abortions, whether therapeutic or voluntary, women reveal feelings of fear and rage related to fantasies of having been anatomically violated. The instrumentation related to evacuation of the uterus may stimulate anguishing and sometimes bizarre fantasies, especially in women who have sadomasochistic dynamics. When the dynamics of baby-as-phallic-compensation are prominent, the sense of being wounded and bleeding may revive archaic castration shock. These women experience abortion as a severe narcissistic injury, and may react with rage and dismay.

CONCLUSION

The central theme of this paper is that the psychosexual meaning of abortion can be understood only if the various types of abortion are distinguished. These include spontaneous abortion, therapeutic abortion either on psychiatric or other medical indications, and voluntary abortion. Furthermore, the meaning of any abortion for any individual can be understood only if that person's developmental level and personality organization are understood. This certainly requires assessment of any psychosexual conflicts important for that individual. It also requires evaluation of the associated level of narcissistic pathology, of the degree to which the fetus has been cathected as a potentially viable person, and of the adaptive flexibility the person has demonstrated in other conflict situations. The contextual aspects of abortion as life crisis have not been stressed in this paper, but interpersonal conflicts about fetal loss and the value systems of important others which are invoked by induced abortion also are extremely important.

The research implications of this analysis are clear. The contradictory findings present in the literature seem to stem from comparisons of dissimilar groups and from failure to distinguish important differences both in types of abortions and in psychological status of women experiencing abortion. What is needed is systematic in-depth data about women and their early pregnancy emotional investment in the anticipated child. Follow-up experience with data gathering within the framework (abortion type by psychosexual level) presented in this paper is also needed to classify abortion experience.

The clinical implications of this analysis can be summarized as a plea for what good psychiatrists always have done—gain an understanding of each woman's personal concerns about abortion in an in-depth assessment, and help guide the patient to understanding of the issues involved.

REFERENCES

Abraham H: New aspects of the psychopathology of patients presenting for termination of pregnancy: Abortion on psychoanalytic grounds. Transactions of the
Topeka Psychoanalytic Society. *Bull Menninger Clin* 33, 1969

Belsey F, Green H S, Lal S, et al: Predictive factors in emotional response to
abortion: King's termination study—IV. *Soc Sci Med* 11: 71-82, 1977

Brewer C: Incidence of post-abortion psychosis: A prospective study. *Br Med J* 1:
476-477, 1977

Burkle F: A developmental approach to post-abortion depression. *Practitioner* 218:
217-225, 1977

Committee on the Working of the Abortion Act (the Lane Commission Report), vol
1. Her Majesty's Stationery Office, 1974

Corney R, Horton F Jr: Pathological grief following spontaneous abortion. *Am J
Psychiatry* 131: 825-827, 1974

Deutsch H: *Psychology of Women,* vol 2. New York, Grune & Stratton, 1945

Drower S, Nash E: Therapeutic abortion on psychiatric grounds, Part 1: A local
study. *South African Mediese Tydskrif* 604-608, 1978a

Drower S, Nash E: Therapeutic abortion on psychiatric grounds, Part 2: The continuing debate. *South African Mediese Tydskrif* 643-647, 1978b

Ewing J, Rouse B: Therapeutic abortion and a prior psychiatric history. *Am J
Psychiatry* 130: 37-40, 1973

Fischer N: Multiple induced abortions—A psychoanalytic case study. *J Am Psychoanal Assoc* 394-497, 1973

Fleck S: Some psychiatric aspects of abortion. *J Nerv Ment Dis* 151: 42-50, 1970

Ford C, Castelnuevo-Tedesco P, Long K: Women who seek therapeutic abortion:
A comparison with women who complete their pregnancies. *Am J Psychiatry*
129: 546-522, 1972

Freud S: The pathogenesis of a case of homosexuality in a woman. *Standard
Edition* 18: 145-172. London, Hogarth Press, 1955

Greenglass E: Therapeutic abortion and psychiatric disturbance in Canadian
women. *Can Psychiatr Assoc J* 21: 453-460, 1976

Group for the advancement of psychiatry: *The Right to Abortion, a Psychiatric
View,* 7, No. 75. Committee on Psychiatry and Law, October 1969

Illsby R, Hall M: Psychosocial aspects of abortion: A review of issues and needed
research. *Bull WHO* 53: 83-106, 1976

Jansson B: Mental disorders after abortion. *Acta Psychiatr Scand* 41: 87-110,
1965

Kane FJ, Ewing J: Therapeutic abortion. *Quo Vadimus Psychosomatics* 9: 202-
206, 1968

Kumar R, Robson K: Previous induced abortion and antenatal depression in
primipara: Preliminary report of a survey of mental health in pregnancy. *Psychol
Med* 8: 711-715, 1978

Lipper S, Feigenbaum W: Obsessive-compulsive neurosis after viewing the fetus during therapeutic abortion. *Am J Psychothe* 30: 666, 1976

Olley P: Age, marriage, personality, and distress: A study of personality factors in women referred for therapeutic abortion. *Semin Psychiatry* 2: 341-351, 1970

Osofsky J, Osofsky H: The psychological reaction of patients to legalized abortion. *Am J Orthopsychiatry* 42 (1) 48, 1972

Patt S, Rappaport R, Barglow P: Follow-up of therapeutic abortion. *Arch Gen Psychiatry* 20: 408–414, 1969

Rosen H: *Therapeutic Abortion,* New York, The Julian Press, 1954

Senay E: Therapeutic abortion. *Arch Gen Psychiatry* 23: 408-415, 1970

Simon NM, Senturia A: Psychiatric sequelae of abortion: review of the literature. *Arch Gen Psychiatry* 15: 378-389, 1966

Spaulding J, Cavenar J: Psychoses following therapeutic abortion. *Am J Psychiatry* 135: 364-365, 1978

Talan K, Kimballc: Characterization of 100 women psychiatrically evaluated for therapeutic abortion. *Arch Gen Psychiatry* 26: 57-577, 1972

Uddenberg N: Reproductive adaptation in mother and daughter. *Acta Psychiatr Scand* (suppl) 254, 1974

Wallerstein JP, Kurtz J, Bar-Din J: Psychosocial sequelae of therapeutic abortion in young unmarried women. *Arch Gen Psychiatry* 27: 828-832, 1972

Warnes H: Delayed after-effects of medically induced abortion. *Can Psychiatr Assoc J* 16: 537-541, 1971

11

Sex Education in Medical Undergraduate Training

William A. Cantrell

HISTORICAL DEVELOPMENT

When one explores the evolution of sex education in medicine, the role of Harold Lief is preeminent. Although his findings were somewhat anticipated in a study of senior medical students and faculty by Greenback (1961), it was Lief (1963) who first documented the ignorance and inexperience of medical students in the sexual domain as compared with their peers. He correlated this discovery with the high incidence—greater than 50 percent—of obsessive-compulsive personality organization in medical students. His studies have been confirmed many times, recently by Marcotte et al. (1977). Later I shall report on our related findings in a medical school population.

In 1968, Harold Lief founded, with support from the Commonwealth Fund, the Center for the Study of Sex Education in Medicine (CSSEM) at the University of Pennsylvania. In 1971, with David M. Reed, he developed the Sexual Knowledge and Attitude Test (SKAT), which was revised in 1972. This instrument has been the major one used to assess sexual attitudes and knowledge of medical students and many other groups. Other dimensions of the SKAT, such as range and variety of sexual experiences, plus biographical data, permit many cross-correlations. The SKAT has now been scored and analyzed for well over 15,000 medical students in the United States and in other countries (personal communication from Dr. Lief).

In the early 1970s Lief and his colleagues at CSSEM held a series of regional workshops for medical educators from many disciplines. Over 90 medical schools sent representatives to these conferences. Many of them in turn became leaders in developing human sexuality courses in their own medical schools

Lief and his associates organized a National Conference on Sex Education in Medicine, held at Airlie House, Virginia, in April 1974. *Sex Education in Medicine,* a book edited by Lief and Karlen, reports the proceedings of that conference. It is the definitive summary of the "state of the art" in the mid-1970s and is an excellent reference source.

In 1960, only three medical schools in the US offered courses in Human Sexuality (Lief and Karlen, 1976). Even in 1968, the year of the founding of CSSEM, only 30 medical schools had such courses. As of 1973, all but 13 percent of US medical schools had formal courses in Human Sexuality; 68 percent of them had courses in the required curriculum. In those schools offering such courses, 88 percent used sexually explicit films as an integral component. Harold Lief has been the prime catalyst behind these profound changes in medical education.

These changes could not have occurred without the influence of many other determinants. The research of Kinsey (1953a, 1953b) and his associates forced us to acknowledge the vast discrepancy between the myth of "normal sexual behavior" in our society and the reality of such behavior. William Masters and Virginia Johnson (1966, 1970), against enormous resistance and even scorn from their medical colleagues, established sexuality as a proper subject for scientific investigation. Meanwhile, profound changes were taking place in the culture at large, the multiple elements of which would be a subject for many years of scientific exploration. Only a few of the important variables will be mentioned. Along with the development of reliable and widely available means of contraception came effective treatment of venereal disease. The decline of moral absolutism and a trend toward secularization of value systems was accompanied by general acceptance of the legitimate rights of women to participate in sex for their own pleasure and not merely for procreation.

Much credit should also be given to medical students of the 1960s and 1970s for their initiative in requesting courses in human sexuality. Tyler (1970) noted the important role of students in development of a sexuality course at the University of Indiana. The author's first efforts in this area followed the urging of members of the graduating class of 1968 of Baylor College of Medicine. They realized they had been taught nothing about sexuality although they would soon be presumed experts by their patients. In response to their request, a series of evening lectures and discussions for the students and their spouses (or significant others) was developed by the author and colleagues. We had no film material available. Like many others who began teaching sexuality under such circumstances, the author would not now choose to teach such a course without audiovisual materials.

Of particular relevance to this paper, a bequest to a Methodist church in San Francisco led to the Glide Foundation, the direct ancestor of the Multimedia Resource Center. Since 1970 this organization has provided medical educators with a large percentage of the films, slides, and other audiovisual materials used in sex education. Their 1980–1981 catalog lists over 80 film titles covering heterosexuality, homosexuality, lesbianism, masturbation, gender identity, bisexual and group sexuality, sexuality for the physically impaired, women's sexuality, sex therapy, massage, and fantasy. (This is only a partial listing.) Another major source of such films is Focus International, Incorporated, of New York City, whose current catalog lists a smaller number of offerings with greater emphasis on sex therapy, counselling, and other aspects of professional skills. A good source of educational films focused on interviewing and counselling is Ortho Pharmaceuticals of Raritan, New Jersey. There are at least half a dozen other sources for such films. In addition, there are many sources of what were formerly called stag films or "hard core pornography." A current euphemism for these is "commercial action films." A complete library of all the reasonably high quality films currently available would cost more than $30,000. Obviously one must be selective to stay within a rational budget.

History of Use of Explicit Films

Paul Gebhard, a collaborator of Alfred Kinsey in the landmark studies of human sexuality and currently Director of the Institute for Sex Research, Inc., Indiana University, Bloomington, states in a personal communication that he and his associates may have been the first to use explicit sex films in teaching medical students. In 1962 they began a seminar for residents, faculty, and some medical students at the Institute for Psychiatric Research, a branch of the Indiana University Medical School. They had a large number of films accumulated by the Institute for Sex Research. Gebhard gave credit to the National Institute of Mental Health for urging him to teach medical students, to the President of Indiana University who released his group from a prior agreement never to teach courses in sexuality, and to Dr. John Nurnberger, then Head of Psychiatry at Indiana University School of Medicine, who strongly supported this teaching. Dr. Edward A. Tyler had attended those early seminars, and in the late 1960s took over the course in human sexuality for medical students. It was introduced in 1968 as an elective and was made a required course the following year (Tyler, 1970). Concurrently, Richard Chilgren at the University of Minnesota, John Money at Johns Hopkins, Herbert Vandervoort at the University of California at San Francisco, and a number of others were developing well-organized, intensive courses in human sexuality. All incorporated films for desensitization, resensitization, and as stimulus material for small group discussions. In 1974 the author reviewed course syllabi from 16 medical schools, representing all geographic regions of this country. The basic design of the courses was remarkably similar except for variability in total course hours. There was nearly equal balance between those courses scheduled over a number of weeks (one or two sessions per week) and those offering a highly concentrated course over a small time period. All but one made extensive use of films and small group discussions along with lectures, educational films, and slides. Several programs included panel discussions involving individuals whose sexual orientations were relatively unfamiliar to students. All these courses were consistent with the ASK (attitudes, skills, knowledge) model (Lief and Karlen, 1976.) Sex educators generally agree that modification of sexual attitudes is the vital component in effective teaching. Knowledge is freely available but will not be meaningfully incorporated into the student's professional identity until an examination of personal attitudes has been facilitated. Acquisition of professional skills is thus promoted.

Goals of Sex Education in Medicine

Perhaps the most comprehensive statement of goals is that of Vandervoort and McIlvenna (1975). They emphasized restructuring of sexual attitude, pointing out the importance of endorsement (giving permission to look and learn about sexuality), acquiring information, learning about patterns of masturbation and homosexual experience, comparison of male and female sexual expression, variants of human sexuality outside the range of the student's own personal experience, desensitization and resensitization, exploration of sexual myths, sexual enrichment, and ultimately development of knowledge and skills to enhance quality of patient care. A more succinct summary is:

Medical sex education should provide information, create attitudes that allow skillful use of the information, and teach skills needed for evaluation, diagnosis, management and referral of sexual and sex-related dysfunctions (Tyler, 1970).

Marcotte and Kilpatrick have stated that "It is neither the province nor the goal of sex education to change students' personal sex attitudes of long years standing; sex education seeks only to help students work more efficiently with their patients." This may be an appropriate statement, but students come to medical school with their own agendas. Often they seek a greater depth of self-understanding and mastery over their own personal anxieties. This is not necessarily an undesirable motivation.

Documentation of Need

In the spring of 1972, the Sexual Knowledge and Attitude Test was administered to all students of a medical school class which had entered in the summer of 1971. The evidence is presented in summary form (Tables 1 and 2). The students were at or about the median for medical students of that year. The range of scores deserves special consideration. Higher scores on the Attitude Scale reflect more liberal attitudes. Higher scores on the Knowledge Scale reflect more correct answers on a true–false test. The highest and lowest scores achieved are almost two standard deviations above or below the mean. The great diversity among students in attitudes, knowledge, and experience makes curriculum planning very difficult. In 1973, the author obtained a sample of SKAT scores from 31 members of the psychiatry faculty at the same medical school. The only area in which the group score of faculty was significantly more "liberal" than that of the students was in the area of autoeroticism. Although the faculty scored somewhat higher in the general knowledge category, the difference was not what one might have hoped and raises troubling questions about psychiatrists as experts on sexuality.

The following material will flesh out the numerical scores of the students: 30 percent of the men agreed or strongly agreed that the spread of sex education is causing a rise in premarital intercourse, as compared to only 6.5 percent of the women. Twenty percent of the men and 18 percent of the women believed possession of contraceptive information was often an incitement to promiscuity. Forty-eight percent of the men and 42 percent of the women believed sexual intercourse should only occur between married couples. Although 53 percent of the men and 48 percent of the women felt men should have premarital intercourse or other sexual experience, only 40 percent of the men and 35 percent of the women felt

TABLE 1. SKAT SCORES

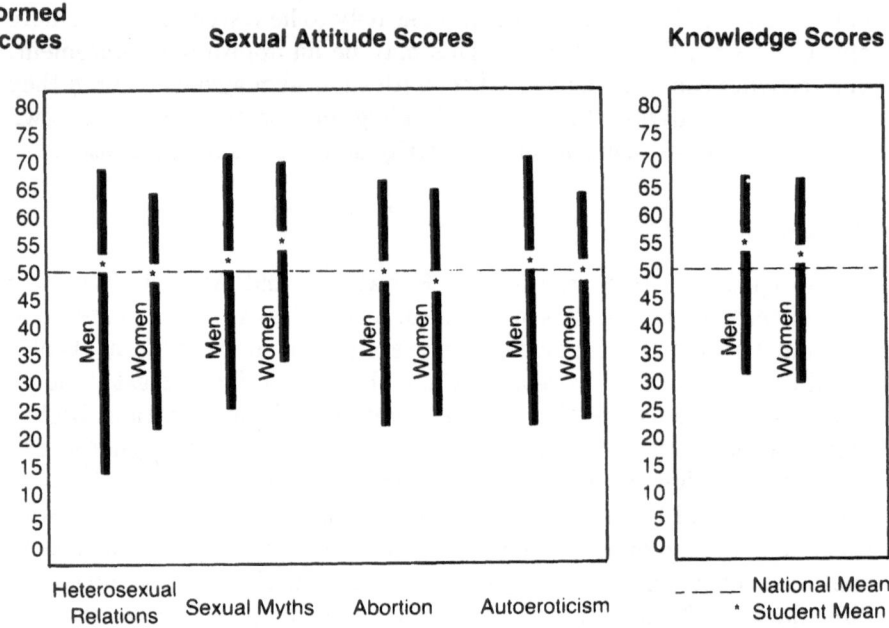

that women should have such experience. Twenty-six percent of the men, as compared to 16 percent of the women, believed our society should encourage virginity among unmarried girls. Surprisingly, 67 percent of men *and* women believed abortion should be available whenever desired by the mother. Seventy-nine percent of both sexes considered masturbation a healthy practice.

Performances on the knowledge scale were slightly above the national norm for men and slightly below for women. About half the class believed transvestites are usually homosexual. Forty-two percent of the men and 55 percent of the women believed that clitoral and vaginal orgasms are physiologically different. In light of the general belief that promiscuity was rampant on college campuses in 1972, it is surprising that half the class thought there was just as much premarital sex a generation ago. Sadly, 60 percent of the men did not know that age affects the sexual

TABLE 2. SKAT ATTITUDE AND KNOWLEDGE SCORES

Scale	Mean	Low	High	Standard deviation
Heterosexual Relations				
TOTAL (N = 174)	50.20	14.17	69.83	11.8
Men (N = 143)	50.79	14.17	69.83	11.9
Women (N = 31)	48.17	21.13	64.61	10.8
Sexual Myths				
TOTAL	50.67	25.44	72.84	10.4
Men	50.22	25.44	72.84	10.4
Women	53.40	34.47	70.59	9.6
Abortion				
TOTAL	48.97	21.73	67.11	10.6
Men	49.28	21.73	67.11	10.5
Women	47.86	23.41	65.43	11.2
Autoeroticism				
TOTAL	51.55	11.02	71.55	10.6
Men	51.74	11.02	71.55	10.9
Women	51.09	23.12	64.29	9.2
Knowledge				
TOTAL (N = 136)	54.22	30.36	68.38	8.3
Men (N = 117)	54.60	30.36	68.38	8.1
Women (N = 19)	51.87	30.36	68.38	9.4

behavior of men more than women. Seventy-one percent of the women and 52 percent of the men believed masturbation to be four times more common in males.

The median age of this class was 23.5 years. 18 percent were women; only 8 percent were nonwhite. The fathers of 65 percent of the class were physicians, other professionals, or executives. Fifty-two percent identified themselves as Protestant, 15 percent Catholic, 12 percent Jewish, and 18 percent "other." Thirty (17 percent) of the students in this sample were or had been married: 26 (18 percent) men and 4 (13 percent) women. Of the never married students, 32 percent of the men and 27 percent of the women had never had sexual intercourse. Nearly 10 percent had never masturbated. In contrast, 24 percent of the men and 13 percent of the women had had more than five different sexual partners.

Half the women and 44 percent of the men rated themselves as definitely liberal in their value systems.

We have data on sexual experience and on the knowledge portion of the SKAT for entering medical school classes of 1973, 1975, 1976, and 1977. The percent of women, blacks, hispanics, and orientals increased significantly.* Patterns of sexual behavior do not appear to be significantly different in any of these subgroups. Many more entering students are either married or have a steady nonmarital sexual partner. In general, the range of sexual activity indicates a significant increase in the percent of students who have had six or more different partners. In fact, our most recent study indicates that this is just as true for women students as for men. Age of onset of masturbatory and partner-related sexual experiences appears to be unchanged for the men but is becoming earlier for the women students. There is more frequent acknowledgement of and acceptance of oral/genital sex as a normal dimension of heterosexual activity. There is also some modest increase in the number of individuals who report experience with group sex. The most significant change in the past seven years is in the area of sexual experiences with a partner of the same sex. This change seems to be more a reflection of changing social mores and a greater willingness of students—on anonymous questionnaires—to acknowledge sexual experiences with same-sex partners. Many more students now enter medical school married or having been married, or having been involved in a continuing nonmarital sexual relationship. Even so, the number of entering students who have never had a sexual partner is in the range of 18 percent. Preliminary evaluation of students never married would indicate that about 25 percent have had no sexual intercourse. Despite this significant shift in the reported range and extent of sexual behavior prior to entering medical school, students performed slightly less well on the Knowledge Scale of the SKAT in the past few years than they did in the early 1970s. Though they have had somewhat earlier exposure to sexual activity, a wider range of sexual activity with a larger number of partners, and a more permissive attitude, they are no more knowledgeable than their counterparts seven years earlier. Furthermore, the range of SKAT scores still reflects great diversity of attitudes and knowledge.

*Women 25 percent; total minority 14 percent.

Diversity of Sexually Explicit Films

In the late 1960s and early 1970s, various sources—notably the Multimedia Resource Center—began producing films depicting various dimensions of human sexual behavior. They were addressed to the larger society, reflecting the rich range of human sexual behavior. Somewhat later, more explicit attention was paid to the needs of physicians and other professionals concerned with sexual dysfunction. Between 1970–1977 a large number of films were produced depicting heterosexual behavior between young and older couples, masturbatory behavior in both sexes, homosexual and lesbian sexual activity, sexual activity involving at least one physically impaired partner, group and bisexual activity. In the late 1970s films designed for use in therapy became widely available.

RESULTS

After more than a decade of experience, it is hard to assess the ultimate impact of sex education on professional skills. It was assumed such instruction would enable students to become more competent in recognizing and treating their patients' sexual problems. It was hoped such training would help physicians direct patients to appropriate sources of help if they did not consider themselves competent to manage the problem. The author is not aware of any study demonstrating such an effect by the strict criteria of scientific research. This lack of documentation on enhancement of professional skills is not unique to sex education. In the current heated debate about mandatory continuing medical education this same issue looms large. Perhaps our assumptions about what comprises good medical training are grounded more in faith than in impeccable statistics.

There is some evidence that a course in human sexuality emphasizing change in attitudes achieves these goals better than courses stressing cognitive information and technical skills. Marcotte and Kilpatrick found that, compared with students who received only lecture/demonstration presentations, students given multimedia presentations including films and group discussions showed significantly greater increments in their SKAT scores (Marcotte and Kilpatrick, 1974).

Chez (1971) reported a study conducted at the University of Pittsburgh during a core clerkship in obstetrics and gynecology. Five explicit films were utilized and were followed by group discussions. One third of the group was at some time bored, repulsed, or surprised. Eighty-one percent of the group were sexually aroused. Sixty-five percent of the students felt the majority of medical students in their class would not be desensitized by the experience but, nevertheless, 82 percent of them felt the session was a worthwhile professional learning experience and recommended its continuation. Gammon and Zisook (1980) reported on a course in sexuality given at the University of Texas at Houston. Of 144 students responding, 93 percent felt sex education should be required of all students. Twenty-two percent of the students rated the course as boring but the authors sensitively pointed out a possible relationship to anxiety arousal. Some students believed current films in the commercial motion picture industry and on television may now do much of the desensitizing that was formerly done by films in sex education courses. Most students rated the group discussions more valuable than the films. Friedman et al. (1978–1979) from the Columbia College of Physicians and Surgeons, report observation of medical students during their exposure to a course in human sexuality including explicit films. They found a significantly greater number of negative responses in male students, largely manifested by overt belligerence, boredom, or going to sleep during the exercise. Even so, the majority of their students rated the course as personally and professionally worthwhile. Elizabeth Stanley (1978) established a course in human sexuality at St. George's Hospital in London. Eighty-six percent of 329 medical students found the course to be personally beneficial and 92 percent thought it professionally beneficial. Dickerson and Myerscough (1979), reporting from the University of Edinburgh, Scotland, found essentially the same student response. Our own surveys of medical students have reflected a similar pattern. A somewhat larger percentage of students always rates the course as *professionally* beneficial as opposed to *personally* beneficial. In our samples, no student has yet indicated that the course was personally harmful. Again, one must wonder about student candor even on anonymous questionnaires.

Whether a course in human sexuality should be required or elective has been debated for the past ten years. We have one sample of students who participated in a concentrated weekend sexual attitude restructuring course after having didactic lecture presentations earlier in the year. We obtained permission from the students to extract their SKAT scores from the larger group. The results indicated that students choosing the elective had previously achieved higher SKAT scores in sexual attitudes and knowledge. This would support the commonly held opinion that elective courses are likely to be passed over by students who need them most.

PROBLEMS IN IMPLEMENTATION

Many US medical schools have doubled the size of entering classes in the past decade. If sex education is enhanced by encouraging spouses and "significant other" partners of students to participate, one is faced with the problem of finding competent group leaders for such a large population. A possible alternative is the inclusion of such courses in clerkships during the clinical years where the numbers of students range from 25–30 on the average. The problem then is one of sustaining motivation for faculty required to repeat such courses six or more times per academic year. The phenomenon of "burnout" is a very real one in this area. Everyone who has taken part in courses in human sexuality knows such an experience is emotionally draining for the teacher.

The example given students in the broader areas of clinical medicine is to a great extent one of emotional detachment and objectivity, with its concomitant emphasis on defense mechanisms of isolation of affect and denial. Teaching human sexuality requires confrontation of these defenses and to some degree their dismantling. If we cannot sustain an appropriate role model in this respect, much of the message will be lost. After the third or fourth exposure to the explicit film material, instructors are prone to become emotionally disengaged. One is reminded of the statement by John Money (1971) that the half life of "pornography" in its ability to elicit sexual arousal and interest is somewhere in the range of two to four hours.

PREDICTIONS FOR THE FUTURE

The author anticipates a greater emphasis in the future on informational material in the area of sexual physiology, more teaching of the etiology and treatment of sexual dysfunction, and diminished use of small group experiences in the pre-clinical years. It is hoped this will be augmented by focused and intensive attitude restructuring experiences at the level of clinical clerkships. Departments of obstetrics and gynecology, departments of urology, departments of pediatrics, departments of family practice, and departments of psychiatry should be particularly attentive to the importance of enriching skills and knowledge relating to sexuality. This is not to say that sexuality is irrelevant to any medical specialty. The initial learning experience of students should be reinforced in the clinical years by teachers who are sensitive and thorough in their assessment of

sexual function. If competence in this area is not perceived as an important skill in the role model teacher, little will be gained.

This sequence cannot be terminated on graduation from medical school.
Unless residency training reinforces the importance of competence in the
area of human sexuality, the ultimate object of our concern—the patient—may benefit little from our efforts.

REFERENCES

Chez RH: Movies of human sexual response as learning aids for medical students. *J Med Educ* 46:977–981, 1971

Dickerson M, Myerscough PR: The evolution of a course in human sexuality—University of Edinburgh, 1972–1978. *Med Educ* 13:432–438, 1979

Friedman RC, Vosburgh GJ, Stern LO: Observed responses of medical students in a sex education seminar on obstetrics and gynecology. *Int J Psychiatry Med* 9:61–70, 1978–1979

Gammon E, Zisook S: Student evaluation of a required sex education course. *J Med Educ* 55:372–375, 1980

Greenback RK: Are medical students learning psychiatry? *Penn Med J* 64:989–992, 1961

Kinsey AC, Pomeroy WB, Martin CE: *Sexual Behavior in the Human Male.* Philadelphia, W. B. Saunders Co, 1953a

Kinsey AC, Pomeroy WB, Martin CE, Gebhard PH: *Sexual Behavior in the Human Female.* Philadelphia, W. B. Saunders Co, 1953b

Lief, HI: What medical schools teach about sex. *Bull Tulane Med Faculty* 22:161–168, 1963

Lief, HI, Karlen A (eds): *Sex Education in Medicine.* New York, Spectrum Publications Inc, 1976

Marcotte DB, Kilpatrick DG: Preliminary evaluation of a sex education course. *J Med Educ* 49:703–705, 1974

Marcotte DB, Kilpatrick DG, Willis A: The Sheppe and Hain study revisited: Professional students and their knowledge and attitudes about sexuality. *Med Educ* 11:201–204, 1977

Masters WH, Johnson VE: *Human Sexual Response.* Boston, Little Brown & Co, 1966

Masters WH, Johnson VE: *Human Sexual Inadequacy.* Boston, Little Brown & Co, 1970

Money J: Pornography and medical education, in Lippard VW (ed): *Macy Conference on Family Planning, Demography, and Human Sexuality in Medical Education.* New York, Josiah Macy Jr. Foundation, 1971, pp 98–109

Stanley E: An introduction to sexuality in the medical curriculum. *Med Educ* 12:441–445, 1978

Tyler EA: Introducing a sex education course into the medical curriculum. *J Med Educ* 45:1025–1030, 1970

Vandervoort HE, McIlvenna T: Sexually explicit media in medical school curricula, in Green R (ed): *Human Sexuality: A Health Practitioner's Text*. Baltimore, Williams and Williams, 1975, pp 234–244

12

Residency Training in Diagnosis and Treatment of Psychosexual Disorders

James W. Lomax

INTRODUCTION

There has been a rapid increase in interest, knowledge, and available treatment approaches to human sexual dysfunction during the past few decades, as reflected in the other chapters in this book. A significant proportion of patients with sexual problems and concerns come to the attention of psychiatrists, and psychiatrists are expected to be knowledgeable and skillful in their disposition. Is this expectation anticipated and met by residency training programs for psychiatrists in the United States?

My involvement in this question began as a Falk Fellow assigned to the American Psychiatric Association's Council on Emerging Issues, one of which was identified as sex education and sex therapy in residency training. This chapter addresses the current state of training in sex education and sex therapy in psychiatry residency, and suggests a model core curriculum.

HISTORICAL CONTEXT

The history of attitudes about sex and sexuality reveals great shifts over time, which Norman Sussman (1976) has outlined in some detail. Sexuality is generally an emotionally charged matter, but the nature of the charge varies widely. In different epochs, sexuality has been condemned as the most evil and undesirable aspect of human existence or idealized as the richest and ennobling of all possible experiences. In the United States we have been heavily influenced by both Puritanical and Victorian traditions. Puritans felt that pleasure in any form diminished one's ability to serve the glory of God. King James I of England had harassed the Puritans, and many of the more staunch believers fled to Holland and then to America's New England coast in the early 1600s. Calvinist principles seemed to develop in this setting even more fully than had been possible in Britain. The Puritans greatly influenced the legal system of the colonies so that laws were passed attempting to regulate sex as a means of procreation without pleasure. These attitudes waxed and waned in ensuing ages, but a resurrection of the Puritan inheritance defined the ambiance of Queen Victoria's reign, occupying almost the entire 19th century. The repressive sexual ethic of that period is viewed by Sussman as an attempt to suppress both the sexual license advocated by the romantic movement and the emerging economic liberation of women stemming from their increased involvement in the labor pool of industrialized nations. The Victorian ethic emphasized the woman's primary responsibility as a wife serving her husband's needs and generated a peculiarly distorted image of the "good woman": delicate, pure, and incapable of sexual feelings. From these influences, a theory of psychological development emerged which clearly and rigidly outlined the marked differences in male and female sexual drives and needs. Efforts to veil evidences of sexuality or anything which might stimulate sexual feelings sometimes reached comic proportions (skirts on table legs, etc). While there were always counter-trends to the Puritanical and Victorian currents, the degree of their continued influence on mainstream American thought is often remarkable.

A weakening of these cultural constraints began after World War I and has steadily continued. One early indication of liberalization was the popular interest in the fiction of F. Scott Fitzgerald and D. H. Lawrence. Both novelists were heavily influenced by psychoanalytic thinking and were not only explicitly interested in sex and sexuality, but described a relationship between the expression of sexual drives or sexual activities and actual health. Such basic changes in attitudes evolved slowly, however. In the 1920s the word sex could not even be mentioned by the public media. The first public birth control centers—evidence of societal recognition of a distinction between sex as a procreative and pleasurable activity—opened during the 1920s, but frequently in clandestine settings and in spite of bureaucratic resistance. The Kinsey reports, *Sexual Behavior in the Human Male* in 1948 and *Sexual Behavior in the Human Female* in 1953, probably represented the first truly scientific inquiry into the descriptive phenomenology of sexuality. Reports such as the book by Kraft-Ebbing had been published earlier. These, however, were characterized by bias and emotionalism, and were often sorely lacking in scientific objectivity. In the 1950s and 1960s, Masters and Johnson greatly expanded our knowledge of normal sexual physiology and behavior and refined the pathophysiology and behavioral pathology of sexual dysfunction. Their work enabled clinicians to assess sexual function based on a systematically developed body of information and paved the way for even more refined scientific methodology, such as sleep laboratory evaluation of impotence. In addition to providing new information about biological parameters, Masters and Johnson demonstrated that many sexual dysfunctions were neither as deep-rooted nor as ominous in their implications as had been predicted by early psychoanalytic investigators. They discovered and documented the success of what Meyer (1976) and others term the "directive sexual therapies." These therapies combine educational and behavioral techniques and, at times, lead to significant functional change following a very short period of treatment.

These contemporary biological and scientific discoveries have occurred in the context of rapid social change. Demands for a broad spectrum of human and civil rights characterized much of the ferment of the 1960s. A social atmosphere developed in which each individual claimed the right to be fulfilled in all parameters of human potential. The parameters where such rights are claimed clearly include sexual function as well as sexual object choice. As might have been predicted, the nearly simultaneous emergence of a large number of individuals demanding the right to experience full sexual satisfaction and a well-advertised collection of easily learned and documentably successful treatment techniques created a marketplace which invited exploitation. Thus, there has been a sudden rise of "clinics" staffed by individuals armed with superficial knowledge about directive sexual therapies and full of promises to deliver the global sort of fulfillment intensely sought, even if dimly conceptualized.

In this context, the physician may often find himself or herself in a rather awkward position. In our culture, physicians—and especially psychiatrists—are viewed as important sources of information about all aspects of life. However, as Lief, and later Woods, have clearly shown, physicians tend to be even more inhibited, less experienced, and less comfortable regarding their sexuality than the majority of their peers. As Cantrell mentions in another chapter in this volume, human sexuality is not taught in that many medical schools, even today. The study to be reported here documents the suspicion that teaching and learning about human sexualities is also far from ideal at the graduate medical education level in a specialty that most Americans very specifically associate with sexual education and treatment of sexual disorders.

RECOMMENDATIONS AND REQUIREMENTS REGARDING SEX EDUCATION AND SEX THERAPY TRAINING IN PSYCHIATRY RESIDENCY

There have been three major conferences on psychiatry residency training in the United States; the proceedings of each have been published in book form (Whitehorn et al., 1953; Eisenberg et al, 1963; Rosenfeld, 1976). These conferences were held in 1952, 1962, and 1975, and therefore represent the viewpoints of psychiatric educators over more than two decades. The report of the 1952 conference does not include the study of sexual function or dysfunction in its hypothetical three-year program, or in its listings of the knowledge, skills, attitudes, and specific subject matter of training in basic or clinical psychiatry. No listings under sexuality or sexual disorders appear in the index of this or the other volumes reporting the proceedings of the three conferences.

The 1962 conference report includes the term "core curriculum." This term is used to describe the "common foundations of basic knowledge" which training programs should give to all residents. Neither human sexuality, sexual disorders, nor related topics are mentioned in the discussion of the core curriculum content or in the listings of subspecialties and special areas of interest to psychiatrists.

In the 1975 conference report there appear for the first time rather detailed outlines of goals and objectives for psychiatry residents at two major programs. However, again, training and education in human sexuality or sexual disorders is mentioned neither by Langsley, McDermott and Enlow in their first postgraduate year objectives, nor by Yager and Pasnau in the sections describing their guidelines and objectives for psychiatry residencies. The volume reporting on this conference has a very sophisticated chapter on goals and values, including a section on the criteria for completion of basic residency education. Human sexuality and sexual disorders are again not mentioned specifically, but there are allusions (without any elaboration) to "recognizing the differences stemming from gender . . . and perception of sex roles."

Another source of learning about what has been expected and required in psychiatry residencies is the "Essentials for Requirements of Approved Residencies in Psychiatry" published in the Directory of Residency Training Programs of the Accreditation Council for Graduate Medical Education (1981). A review of books for the years 1965, 1975, and 1981 fails to show any mention of any requirement regarding human sexuality or sexual disorders in an approved residency program. One might stretch the requirement regarding "providing an understanding of physical and psychological development" to include development of sexuality and sexual function, but this is certainly not an explicit component.

There are some indicators, however, that residency training directors consider that information about human sexual and psychosexual disorders should be included in the core curriculum of residency training. In his book, *A Resident's Guide to Psychiatric Education*, Michael Thompson (1979) includes psychosexual disorders in the items listed as terminal and enabling objectives for psychiatry residency. Thompson believes that the resident should "be able to relate the onset and recurrence of deviant behavior to predisposing factors and important life conflicts of the individual . . . and be able to discuss treatment approaches commonly used in the management of psychosexual disorders, such as psychotherapy, behavior therapy, and the techniques popularized by Masters and Johnson." Bowden, Humphrey, and Thompson (1980) did a survey of psychiatry residency training directors and developed a list of items which were considered to be essential by at least 50 percent of the educators participating in the survey. Three items related to sexuality and sexual disorders are in this list: knowledge of the effect of illness and medication on sexual behavior, knowledge of treatment approaches for sexual deviations, and the ability to compare male and female life cycles regarding achievement, motivation, affiliation, and sexuality.

SURVEY OF PSYCHIATRY RESIDENCY DIRECTORS

In 1978, the author undertook a survey of psychiatry residency directors as a member of the American Psychiatric Association Task Force on Sex Education and Sex Therapy, chaired by Edward Auer, MD. The survey was done as part of the function of that task force, but this report represents only the views of this author. The survey was an attempt to determine what material regarding sex education and sex therapy is being taught in U.S. residency programs, by what means it is taught, where it is taught, the nature of opportunities for applying information learned about sex education and sex therapy, how competency for sex education and sex therapy is assessed and documented, what is taught about ethical issues in relation to sex education and sex therapy, and, finally, to obtain a general statement from each program regarding a conceptual approach to sexual problems. The questionnaire was distributed to all institutional members of the American Association of Directors of Psychiatry Residency Training Programs (AADPRT). This group of psychiatric educators was chosen because of the ready access to its membership list and the observation that this group is often polled on matters of residency education and seems disposed to respond to such questionnaires. The questionnaire was sent to 150 institutional members of the AADPRT; there were 96 responses (64 percent of those polled). Eighty of the responding programs (83 percent) indicated that the material regarding sex education and sex therapy was presented in some form by their program. Educational methods were divided between lectures, films, videotapes, and seminars. Many programs used two or more of those methods. In only 12 programs, however, was there a subspecialty assignment which emphasized sex education and sex therapy as part of a required curriculum. The number of didactic sessions devoted to sex education and sex therapy ranged from 0–52 sessions, with an average of about 10.5. The total number of hours devoted to the material ranged from 0–115, with an average of 17 hours per resident.

One quarter of the residency programs which responded had no opportunity for clinical or professional activities in either sex education or sex therapy within their structure. Only 18 programs (19 percent) had opportunities for residents to teach sex education. Two thirds of the programs had some opportunity for their residents to treat patients with sexual dysfunction, and one fourth had a specific affiliated sexual dysfunction clinic (but only 10 percent offered this clinic as a training elective).

Supervisors with expertise in sex education or sex therapy are scarce. Only one-third of the programs have more than two supervisors with this special interest. Eighty-five percent of the programs use psychiatrists for supervision, but a wide variety of other professionals teach in these settings: obstetricians, gynecologists, registered nurses, psychologists, chaplains, and other educators. The main form of supervision is in the traditional one-to-one format, but 19 programs use direct observation of clinical skills either through a two-way mirror or by videotape.

Systematic assessment of the resident's competence in sexual therapy, teaching, and associated ethical issues is reported by only a small minority of residency programs. Thirteen programs administer a specific written examination, and eight programs utilize direct observation of clinical skills to test the resident's knowledge and skills in managing sexual issues. Another four programs assign specific supervisors to determine competence in sex education and sex therapy, but the methods used in this determination were not specified. Only 37 of the programs deal directly with ethical issues in sexual therapy and sex education. Another 16 programs reported that they did not specifically deal with the ethics of sexual therapy but included this topic in the broad scope of teaching activities. Issues which were felt to require specific attention included clarity about personal values of the therapist and patient, avoidance of patient/therapist contact in a physical or sexual sense, interdisciplinary teaching, and the importance of including religious considerations in ethical discussions. A few programs also include topics such as countertransference issues, confidentiality and informed consent, medical-legal issues, and the use of surrogates. One program utilizes the Eastern Association of Sexual Therapists' Ethical Code.

This group of residency educators does not feel that sexual education and sexual therapy can be taught as an isolated behavior or behavioral abnormality. Only 5 percent of the programs reported that their general approach was that sexual dysfunction represents an isolated behavioral symptom. In contrast, 44 percent of the programs indicated that their general approach was psychodynamic or interpersonal, and another 50 percent indicated that dynamic, interpersonal, and isolated behavioral symptom models were all helpful, depending upon individual cases. The only specific conceptual model mentioned was that of Helen Kaplan.

RECOMMENDATIONS

It appears that even among the very best adjusted and happily married individuals, there is a significant incidence of sexual difficulties. This incidence is undoubtedly greater in the population of individuals who seek psychiatric consultation. Psychiatrists should therefore be interested in these problems, should be comfortable in working with them, and should be prepared to deal effectively with them. Their specialty training should prepare them for this. Psychiatry residency education should enable the graduate to identify and treat sexual disorders and to know the range of normal expression of human sexuality. The core curriculum of psychiatry residency programs should include at least the didactic and experiential exercises which would make this possible. For those who wish to become competent as sex therapists, residency programs should provide additional didactic information, as well as a supervised clinical setting for supervised experience in the evaluation and treatment of sexual problems.

All psychiatry residency programs should specify as a terminal objective that the graduating psychiatrist: (1) demonstrate knowledge of the prevalence of sexual problems, (2) demonstrate knowledge of the normal development and expression of sexuality in both men and women, (3) demonstrate knowledge regarding the nature of sexual object choice, (4) demonstrate knowledge of the effects of prescribed and OTC medications and alcohol on sexual function, (5) demonstrate knowledge of effective treatment alternatives for sexual disorders, (6) be able to perform a thorough sexual history, (7) be able to successfully refer patients with sexual problems to appropriate treatment resources, and (8) demonstrate awareness of ethical considerations associated with treatment of sexual disorders.

The rather minimal level of training in human sexuality and human sexual disorders revealed by this survey makes it probable that these goals are not being met. Undoubtedly, many patients' sexual questions and problems are not dealt with or are overlooked because of the psychiatrist's ignorance or discomfort.

To insure that a psychiatry resident acquires special competence in the treatment of sexual dysfunctions, he or she should have had a supervised clinical experience in the evaluation and treatment of sexual disorders in addition to the basic training just described. This training should include supervised treatment using behavioral therapy and couples or family therapy in addition to the directive sexual therapies.

CONCLUSION

Graduates of psychiatry residency programs in the United States will inevitably encounter substantial numbers of patients with significant sexual disorders. These physicians will find themselves in the position of being looked to as important sources of information, experts in human sexuality. Psychiatric education has traditionally approached sexuality from an intrapsychic, psychodynamic orientation with an emphasis on the very personal significance of early sexual experiences and fantasies—infantile sexuality, oedipal situation, etc. Lay perception of psychiatrists varies widely if not wildly with regard to theoretical and even personal issues surrounding sexuality. An increasing percentage of the general public is aware that new knowledge exists regarding epidemiology, physiology, and treatment of sexual disorders. Psychiatrists are consulted by individuals who believe that their physician will be able to evaluate and treat an increasingly broad spectrum of sexual complaints. This consultation will be awkward and inappropriate if the psychiatrist has had no exposure to sex education or sex therapy in the specialty residency. We need to insure a more predictable educational experience for our residents, as well as better documentation of their competence in knowledge and skills related to human sexual function and dysfunction. Psychiatry and psychiatrists have a unique perspective to bring to sex education and sex therapy. Special skills and training in the psychodynamics of human behavior should be supplemented by experiences in the core curriculum of residency training, which will develop the psychiatrist's ability to manage sexual dysfunction. The terminal objectives proposed here for the core curriculum of psychiatry residencies would meet these needs.

REFERENCES

Accreditations Council on Graduate Medical Education: Essentials of Requirements for Approved Residencies in Psychiatry. *Directory of Residency Training Programs.* Chicago, American Medical Association, 1981, pp 45–49

Bowden C, Humphrey G, Thompson M: Priorities in psychiatric residency training. *Am J Psychiatry*137(10):1243–1246, 1980

Eisenberg L, Farnsworth D, Garber R, et al (editorial board): Training psychiatrists to meet changing needs. *Proceedings of the 1962 American Psychiatric Association Conference,* Washington, DC, 1963

Lief HI: Sexual attitude and behavior of medical students: implications for medical practice, In Noch E, Jessner L, Abse D (eds): *Marriage Counseling in Medical Practice.* Chapel Hill, University of North Carolina Press, 1964

Meyer JK: Training and accreditation for the treatment of sexual disorders. *Am J Psychiatry* 33(4):389–394, 1976

Rosenfeld A (ed): Psychiatric education: Prologue to the 1980s. *Report of 1975 American Psychiatric Association Conference.* Washington DC, 1976

Sussman N: Sex and sexuality in history, In Sadoch B, Kaplan H, Freedman A (eds): *The Sexual Experience.* Baltimore, Williams and Wilkins, 1976, pp 7–70

Thompson MGG: *A Resident's Guide to Psychiatric Education.* New York, Plenum Press, 1979

Whitehorn J, Graceland F, Lippard V, Malamud W: The psychiatrist—his training and development. *Proceedings of the 1952 American Psychiatric Association Conference.* Washington, DC 1953

Wood SM, Natterson J: Sexual attitudes of medical students: Some implications for medical education. *Am J Psychiatry* 124:323-332, 1967

Index